UP FROM THE ASHES

UP FROM THE ASHES

There is Life After a Stroke

By James A. Young, C.A.P.

The Inner Path Publishing Corp.
Sarasota, FL

© 1995 by James A. Young

All rights reserved. No part of this book shall be reproduced, stored in a retrieval system, or transmitted by any means, electronic, mechanical, photocopying, recording, or otherwise, without written permission from the publisher.

Cover copyright © 1997 by James A. Young

Publisher's Cataloging in Publication

Young, James A.
Up From the Ashes : There Is Life After A Stroke.
/ James A. Young

Includes bibliographical references.

1. Healing. 2. Mind and body. 3. Self-help. 4. Health.
5. Psychology. 6. Spirtuality. 7. Holistic medicine.

ISBN: 0-9651506-0-7

A DEDICATION...

MY LOVE AND APPRECIATION

TO GINGER DANIEL.

TO MY DAUGHTERS, KATIE, TAMMIE, AND LAURIE.

TO LUCY AND TIGER.

TO PEG BUZZELLI

THANK YOU FOR YOUR DREAM

IT WORKS IF YOU WORK IT!

WITHOUT ALL OF YOU, I DON'T KNOW IF I COULD HAVE

MADE IT.

I AM FOREVER GRATEFUL.

ACKNOWLEDGMENTS

Ginger Daniel, who went to hell and back with me. I love you. Laurie Young, who supported me through my struggle, helped me to drive again, helped me create my living situation, and supported me through the writing of this book. Katie Young, who took over in the beginning and made it possible to get some help from the State and Social Security Disability and supported me throughout my struggle. Tammie Golabek, who helped with the paperwork which made it possible to get some help from the state and Social Security Disability, and also gave me support throughout my struggle and helped with typing. My sister Shirley and her family for their support. My brother Ron and his family, for their support. Margaret Scripps Buzzelli, who made it possible for me to go to biofeedback training, for straightening out my insurance, and for support throughout my struggle to get well. George Rozelle, Ph.D. and Thomas H. Budzynski, Ph.D. who worked with me three times a week for a year, doing Biofeedback training and Light and Sound therapy. Chris Pantzis, who gave me support and helped with the insurance papers. Anabasis Staff, for all your support. John Heider and Andrew Babiak, for your guidance and support in getting me up and walking again. Home Health Service Staff, for the nurses, and "Teach," Phyllis H. Joseph MS. C.C.C., Speech Language Pathology. The male nurse on staff June 20, 1992 day shift; thank-you for your compassion and that of Hospital and Doctors. Cindy Ann Yenchko, who wrote the poem "Up From the Ashes." Kathleen Carrillo (Marcus), who helped me to get in touch with my artist self. Andrew Marcus, who worked with me, and on me through acupuncture. Dorothy Magby, the goddess in the garden. The fellowship of the program of Alcoholics Anonymous. My deepest appreciation to Walton Beacham and Deborah Beacham for their unselfish editorial guidance and enthusiastic encouragement. Thanks to my many clients and to all the extras in my drama. You are all truly loving, giving beings.

Contents

A DEDICATION..v
ACKNOWLEDGMENTS..vii
FOREWARD...xi
PREFACE..xv
Chapter 1   DEATH..7
Chapter 2   THE HERO'S JOURNEY...................................15
Chapter 3   BEGINNING OF THE STRUGGLE....................21
Chapter 4   JOURNEY TO HELL..41
Chapter 5   SOCIAL SECURITY..45
Chapter 6   OH, NO, NOT THE TRAILER!..........................47
Chapter 7   THE TRIP..49
Chapter 8   EXPRESSION...53
Chapter 9   THE PSYCHIC SURGEON................................55
Chapter 10   BIOFEEDBACK..59
Chapter 11   THE CAMPING TRIP......................................65
Chapter 12   THE BREAKUP..71
Chapter 13   THE GOURD LADY..75
Chapter 14   A HOME FOR ME..79
Chapter 15   SEARCHING FOR A NEW SELF......................87
Chapter 16   BROKEN WING..101
Chapter 17   THE ACUPUNCTURE AND HERB DOCTORS....105
Chapter 18   THE WRITER..109
Chapter 19   THE BRIDGE..113
Chapter 20   REBIRTH..119
Chapter 21   SPIRIT IS THE ANSWER TO SEPARATION...127
Chapter 22   TRAGEDY or BLESSING?.......................129
AFTERWORD..135
INFORMATION AND SOURCES...137
FROM THE AUTHOR! BOOK COVER STORY....................141
ABOUT THE AUTHOR...145

FOREWARD

I still remember that balmy Florida afternoon when I first saw my former professional colleague walk into the room. Actually, it was more like a shuffle, not at all like the spirited gait to which I was accustomed. We, the staff of Anabasis, a human potential retreat, were in the midst of our weekly process group when Jim returned to the site of some of his extraordinary work with people in distress. Now, this dedicated servant was clearly the one in distress.

As he carefully placed his uncooperative body on the couch and struggled to spit out a few words of greeting, I saw a mere shadow of the man I knew and admired. Through, as we all knew, suddenly and without warning, he had been stricken with a debilitating stroke. I also saw that indomitable spirit that had carried him through a lifetime of challenges. It was also hard to overlook the anger and frustration he was feeling over the failure of the healthcare system to attend to his emotional needs and preserve his dignity. Though prompt medical intervention had probably saved his life, and certainly prevented further damage, the system had somehow failed him.

As Jim proceeded to tell us about his anguish, his fears, his depression, and the gamut of human emotions that accompanied him through his rehabilitation process, I realized that I could only remotely understand what it was like to suffer a stroke. As he continued, it became clear that the caring professionals that were trained to help him didn't really understand either. As I painfully listened to him search for the words he wanted, then make several attempts to articulate the words, and often come out with the wrong words, I didn't know how to respond. Should I help him find the words? Should I finish sentences for him? Should I just let him struggle? Should I speak loudly, slowly, carefully enunciating each word? Would that be demeaning to him?

Sensing that others now regarding him to be mentally, as well as physically incapacitated, some bordering on condescending, I, like others in the room, tried to relate to Jim as we always had. I somehow knew his damaged brain could still think quite clearly, but the wiring for expressing those thoughts had many broken circuits. I admired his account of his valiant attempts to make the helpers listen to him. Even more, I admired his courageous attempt to rehabilitate himself. How frustrating it must have been for a man, trained to attend to people's emotional needs, to find his own feelings often ignored by those who were more concerned with fixing his body.

What could I do to help my friend? Anabasis had evolved out of addictions treatment into human potential work. Guided by the vision of Peg Buzzelli, we were committed to the research and development of innovations in the exploration and development of the sense of self. It was in this spirit that I had studied an emerging new science/art with exciting potential. It was called neurofeedback, or neurotherapy, or EEG biofeedback. By any name, it offered a new way to help people help themselves. I had enjoyed remarkable success with alpha/theta brain wave training for addictions and I had begun to learn about other applications of the technology, including stroke rehabilitation. By learning to suppress irregular slow wave theta activity, a product of the injured brain, and augmenting beta, or fast wave activity, a signature of the functional state, one could apparently guide the brain into an accelerated and enhanced healing process, above and beyond what otherwise might be possible with more conventional approaches.

At the time Anabasis had added the biofeedback-based research and development project under my direction. We had brought in Dr. Tom Budzynski, a pioneer in biofeedback research, to assist us in this effort. With our combined interest in neurotechnology and involvement in the field, we had access to the latest neurofeedback equipment and experimental applications. Within this foundation, Jim's case presented an excellent opportunity to not only help a fallen colleague, but also to make a contribution to the clinical applications of this new technology. When I discussed with Jim the idea of participating in a research study he jumped at it with both feet.

As the principal investigator in this case study, I had many questions. As the subject, Jim provided many of the answers. I listened and learned. And Jim, after having neurologically stabilized one year after the stroke, suddenly began to make great strides. To our amazement and delight, his facilitates of communication were coming back. We continued the project for about a year and Jim was back. He was flying again, albeit a little more slowly. I don't know how much I helped Jim, but I do know how much I learned from him. Today, I am using that knowledge to help other stroke survivors. Even when they are completely aphasic, I can understand them.

I encouraged Jim to write this book for two reasons. The writing process itself was, I believe, very therapeutic. But, on a grander scale, herein is a message that needs to be delivered, a story that needs to be told, a text that needs to be read by healthcare workers, survivors of stroke and their loved ones. The very existence of this manuscript is a testament to the resilience of the human brain and the power of the human spirit.

George R. Rozelle, Ph.D.
Psychotherapist, Neurotherapist, and Friend

PREFACE

The story you are about to read is a true story, though at times it will seem to you unbelievable, as it is to me now. If I were reading this story, I would say this is a figment of a very imaginative person. I was like you before all this happened to me; and now I can only relate to you a chain of miracles, each link formed by almost unfathomable events. Believe it all. It is my deepest truth, which I have no choice but to tell you, I am the Ancient Mariner, returned from the depths. I haunt myself with the mirror. I am fixed by my own eye.

This is a story about "POWER" that embodies the opposites, powerless/power, conscious/unconscious, ego/spirit, dark/light, death/life, male/female, fear/peace, to mention a few. They collide and struggle with one another, in an attempt to give birth to psyche wholeness. The spirit is then born out of the conflict of the opposites, the spirit then assumes its rightful place as the center of the psyche, reconciling the psyche into a new and harmonious whole.

A stroke was the instrument that assaulted my being, altering the course and quality of my life. My whole being was shattered on a physical, emotional, mental, and spiritual level. I was like "Humpty Dumpty"—all the kings horses, all the kings men, couldn't put me together again.

Conventional medical interventions contributed to my anguish. Their treatment seemed to focus on preparing me to be a stroke victim, rather than a fully functioning, integrated human being.

The lack of power was my dilemma. I needed to find a power greater than my Ego, to rise from what was seeming death and hopelessness to life! I was imprisoned between two worlds. In this position, it required me to make some choices. I chose the quest for wholeness, I knew that it would require a radical shift in focus of awareness, from external to internal, tapping into my inner resources. I chose numerous innovative alternative methods to help me in my quest.

Only I could map the path of myself, taking my bearing, charting my experiences. I have only the gift of sharing, I cannot share my experience, only to tell about them in hopes that they can help you on your own journey. I also hope that it will support and encourage your own aspirations, while tapping into your inner resources.

This story is for everyone, written especially for those who are experiencing stroke recovery, and anyone who has any disease, affliction, or who is confronted with insurmountable life obstacles.

I invite everyone to come with me on my inner journey, into my physical, emotional, mental, and spiritual bodies. My truth is hidden deep within.

We will travel between worlds of concrete and abstract form.

"I MUST SHAPE MY LIFE OUT OF MYSELF —
OUT OF WHAT MY INNER BEING TELLS
ME, OR WHAT NATURE BRINGS TO ME."

— Carl Jung

UP FROM THE ASHES
By
Cindy Ann Yenchko
Part 1

Birth, Death, Rebirth
All fragments of one
Interweaving to make whole
Through a black vastness arrives
only to find uncertainty
on the other side

Cold, Helpless, Alone . . .
at the hands of others
If only to grasp the innocence of youth
that was boarded and closed
to anyone wanting to enter
Except to the mask
of death . . .

Alone . . . Again
the suit of Armor stands to watch
as if keeping guard
Helpless and Merciless
I too am forced to watch in elevation
the immense grief and suffering
of my poor soul's defenselessness

UP FROM THE ASHES
Part 2

Gripping sanity
by a mere thread
I am conscious of my responsibility
Trapped in this Abyss
by an unsure assailant
I am sentenced to Death

My agenda warfare
though engulfed in the smoldering remains
of what Once was . . .

Arise, I command
from beneath the Stygian hue
Resurrected—I emerge
Again . . . Alone
but . . .

UP FROM THE ASHES

Chapter 1

DEATH

On Friday, June 19, 1992, I had no idea that my whole life as I knew it would change.

My girlfriend Ginger and I were visiting her mother on Fort Myers beach. All week I felt very tired. I attributed this to my being overworked. I had started a private counseling practice, while I was also counseling full time at a treatment center. We were at Ginger's mother's beach house to rest and relax.

On this particular day we decided to go out for dinner. Ginger was driving her mother's car. Her mother was in the front and I was in the back. As we were driving to the restaurant, we passed the new hospital. I felt a strange feeling come over me. I kept looking at the hospital as though I were in a trance. As we passed it, I turned around, continuing to look at it. I felt a knot in the pit of my stomach. The hospital seemed to be beckoning to me as I felt its coldness, like death was smiling at me and it sent chills throughout my body. It was like a dream that faded as quickly as it had come.

We arrived at the restaurant. They seated us at a table that had a view of the grounds. It was peaceful looking out into the garden with its beautiful trees and flowers. In the background was a piano player, playing a peaceful tune. We ordered our food, proceeding to talk about a number of subjects. I was feeling relaxed and was really enjoying myself. The meal came. It was superb. I was feeling great, when all of a sudden in my body, I felt a strange reaction. I sensed something was wrong. I became nervous, my anxiety level rose. I had to go to the men's room. I didn't know what was happening to me, so I blocked my thoughts and feelings. This seemed to calm me down. I went back to the table to eat a piece of pie. As I was eating, my fork flew out of my hand and flew across the room. I turned to see where it went, people were turning to look at me and I felt embarrassed. Ginger looked at me, as if to say "What are you doing? Are you nuts?" My anxiety level quickly shot back up again, so I quit eating and lit a cigarette to relax.

I put the cigarette in my mouth, taking a puff. All of a sudden the cigarette flew out of my hand and across the room. Ginger looked at me again. I thought to myself, "We better get out of here before I burn the building down." I couldn't understand what was happening to me. Apparently Ginger got the message. While we were waiting for the check, my anxiety level hit its highest peak. All I could think to do was to run.

We left the restaurant. I was relieved to be out of there. Ginger was still driving. I was in the back seat. We were on our way back to the beach. When we were about one hundred yards from the entrance to the hospital, my whole right side felt as though it was paralyzed. I said, "Ginger! My whole right side is numb." Those were the last words out of my mouth. I was mute. At that moment I was terrified. We were right in front of the hospital, Ginger sped up the drive, right to its entrance. We went right to the emergency room. I couldn't talk. I was trying to feel my right side with my left hand. I wanted to see if my right side was missing. They came with a wheelchair and wheeled me into the emergency room and they put me on a bed. I was fully conscious, in fact my mind was very clear. My anxiety seemed to disappear. I felt a sensation, even though I was lying down. It was like I was multidimensional. I was able to look from a higher level and see in four directions at the same time.

I just lay there and watched. I was in a large open room. There was a woman in another bed sobbing. Ginger was by my bed, a nurse was checking my blood pressure, a doctor was checking me over, then it seemed like they all left. I watched two different nurses walk by, I felt invisible and the place seemed deserted. I had no idea of what had happened to me. As I was looking at myself, I was wondering if I were dead. Yet I could see my body breathing and stirring. Why isn't someone doing something for me. I wasn't frightened, nor did I feel any discomfort. I looked at the clock. I felt like I was lying there for hours. Finally someone came and pushed my bed down the hall and into a room. I didn't know what they were going to do. No one seemed to want to talk to me. They did a CAT scan and an echocardiogram cardiac doppler. Then, they pushed me to a patient room. They put an IV needle in my wrist and hooked it to a bag. Then they wired my chest, to monitor my EKG. Still no one talked to me. I thought, "Maybe everything is okay and I'll be able to get out of here in the morning." I felt all alone. Ginger came into the room and talked to me. It seemed as if I couldn't grasp what she was saying. I wanted to talk but nothing would come out of my mouth. She stayed a while. Her mother had been in the waiting room and she had to leave. She kissed me, and touched me in a way that felt assuring. The room was freezing. I had worked in hospitals for twenty five years, yet I had never been a patient. I had joked many times over the years, "Don't get sick on Friday evening, because they put you in a freezer until Monday morning, when they can check your insurance." My mind was searching, wanting to know what had happened to me. My body seemed frozen, I began to shake and tremble. I felt a strong sense of abandonment coupled with terror. On a deep level, I sensed that the hospital would kill me, so I had a strong urge to run, but I couldn't. There I was, trapped. It was as if my whole being, on a physical, emotional, mental, and spiritual level was being pulled apart.

Then I was looking down at my body. My body was encased in a black suit of armor. I felt at peace, free, and with no fear. As I looked down behind the armor, my eyes were moving back and forth, they were full of fear. As I was hovering over my body, I knew intuitively that I had suffered massive damage. I could see a black area in my left brain. It looked like burnt ash. My body was cold and my mind was trying to understand what was happening to me. Something in my memory surfaced. It was that the soul will leave the body, usually in reaction to a traumatic event. It's called soul loss. It's the way the psyche of a person can survive a painful event. It was a long lonely, sleepless night.

Throughout the night, one of the wires going to my chest kept falling off. The night nurse would come in and spew his anger and frustration on me. After awhile I felt guilty. I thought, "Doesn't anyone here have any compassion?" My question had been answered. The day nurse came in, I could feel his compassion. He sat on the edge of the bed and supported me while allowing me to cry. I felt grateful. Then he left.

My mind was searching, like a giant computer. I wondered why I didn't die. I felt dead, abandoned, and powerless. I didn't know what had happened to me.

My thoughts took me back to last night's experience. It was not strange to me because of my past experiences in death and rebirth. I could see my egos' eyes, they were full of fear. He was trying to protect himself with a suit of armor. I could see my soul, feeling freedom. The balance between freedom and responsibility.

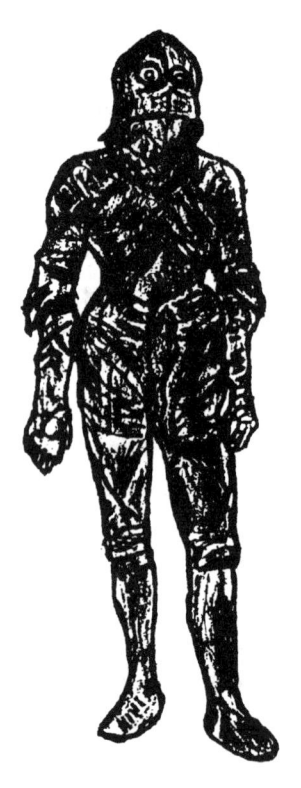

My thoughts came back to the moment. I didn't know if I could get up. How were my needs going to be met? I couldn't speak. I didn't want to be in this condition. How could I get out of this world? I didn't have anything to kill myself with. I was frustrated and angry. I wished I were dead.

Ginger came to see me. She had called my daughters and two of them were on their way to Fort Myers. I initially reacted negatively, thinking that I would only be here for a few days and then everything will be okay. As Ginger continued talking to me, I felt like I wasn't there. I was conscious, I could see her talking, I could hear her voice, but her words weren't registering in my brain. I knew she said something about my daughters, but nothing else. My thoughts seemed separate from my brain and body. It was like I was in another dimension, all alone trapped between worlds. Ginger had to leave for awhile. My mind went back to searching. It was like a tape player that I controlled, fast forward, and rewind, it went back and forth. Nothing is independent, everything is in some way related to something.

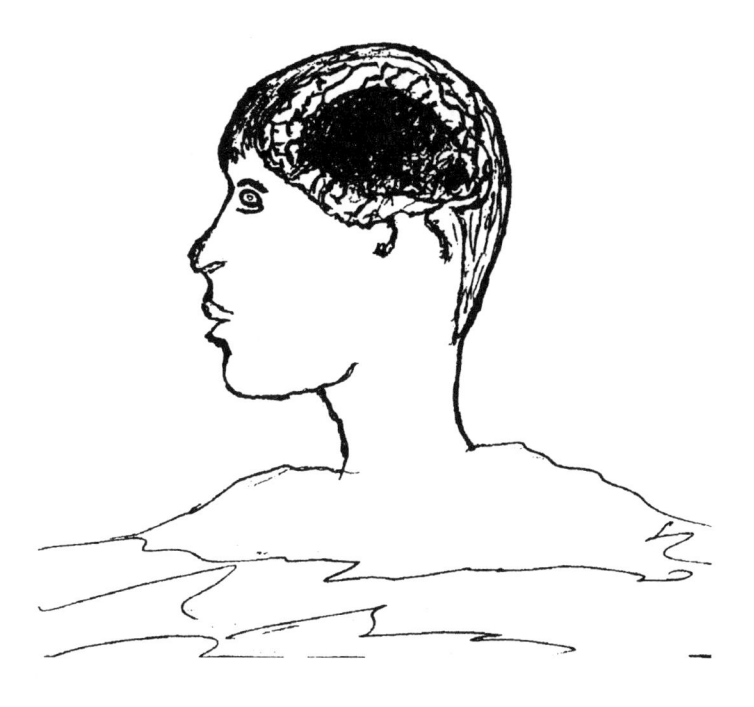

My mind went back to twenty-five years ago when I had just come off drinking. When I had detoxified myself, I went into a treatment center for alcoholism. The second day in treatment, I had what I considered to be a spiritual experience. I was in bed. It was a bright sunny day, all of a sudden everything went black. I was lying there in this darkness with no thoughts or feelings. I was in total peace. Then all of a sudden a ray of bright light shone on my hand, moving to surround my body. I felt a soothing touch, and I knew at that moment that I didn't have to drink ever again. I felt feelings of ecstasy. From that day on, I never had the urge to drink again.

I also began to remember the time when I was about eight years old and a neighbor kid and myself were on the rocks below the dam. We knew that we had ten minutes to get off the rocks if they opened the gates. We would go to the farthest point, then run back across the rocks, timing ourselves, to see if we could get back before the gates opened. There were pools of water in the rocks. We called two of them little punch and big punch, because they looked like punch bowls. Big punch was deep and the sides were slippery. My buddy was heavy and fat, while I was a little runt. He fell into big punch. Intuitively I jumped into save him. I came behind him, he turned and grabbed me pulling me under the water. I couldn't get my head above the water. I struggled until I was exhausted. At that moment I went limp. I felt peaceful, then I felt a surge of energy rush into my body. I was able to grab onto a rock. I came up and out of the water with my buddy still hanging onto me. Then I collapsed, feeling totally exhausted. At thirteen and also again at eighteen, I was involved with drowning, from which I was rescued. Both times I felt at peace, surrounded by blackness. What could all of this mean?

Then my mind went to the story of "Anabasis," written by Xenophon, an ancient Greek historian. He tells how in 401 B.C., he marched with an army of Greek warriors into Asia Minor to overthrow the King of Persia. They were defeated in battle. Leaderless and surrounded by the enemy, the Greeks appeared destined for death or slavery. Xenophon met the panicked, dispirited troops in council and challenged them to become their own generals and devise a strategy to survive. Inspired by his challenge, the Greeks rediscovered their strength. Eighty percent of them heroically made it to their homeland.

I then remembered the movie, "The Other Side of the Mountain." Specifically "the decision" to get up and walk.

I didn't want to be a victim. At this point, I was in shock. This shock lasted fifteen months. It would become a process of letting go. I still did not realize the extent of my damage. Although there were people there to support me, I felt alone, lost, afraid, confused, and disoriented. I knew I had to walk. This was my first priority.

The words of Xenophon were fresh in my mind, "Challenged," "Be my own general," "Devise a strategy." Then I was amused, when I realized I was a general for the last twenty-five years, helping alcoholics and drug dependents to get their shattered lives together.

My mind went into my own alcoholism. I ran a parallel with my alcoholism and my stroke. My feelings now, are the same as twenty-five years ago. When I was drunk, I couldn't walk or talk. When I detoxed, I felt alone, lost, afraid, confused, and disoriented. Then a vision of the "Big Book of Alcoholics Anonymous" flashed into my mind. I saw Chapter 5, "How It Works"

> Rarely have we seen a person fail who has thoroughly followed our path. If you have decided and are *willing to go to any length to get it*—then you are ready to take certain steps. We thought we could find an easier, softer way, but we could not. With all earnestness at our command, we beg of you to be fearless and thorough from the very start. Without help, it is too much for us. But there is One who has all power—That one is God. May you find him now! Half measures availed us nothing. We stood at the turning point. We asked His protection and care with complete abandon.

Here are the steps we took, which are suggested as a program of recovery:

1. That I am powerless and can't manage my life.
2. That probably no human power could relieve my condition. That God could and would if he were sought.
3. Made a decision to turn my will over to the care of God as we understood Him.

This will be the beginning of my Hero's Journey.

Chapter 2

THE HERO'S JOURNEY

For me (the hero) to live, I must fight and sacrifice my longing for the past. Only then will I be able to rise to new heights. I must climb to the peaks of my aspirations, one step at a time. By placing one foot in front of the other, I will reach the summit of the highest mountain.

I sensed that if I didn't get out of bed now, I would never be able to get out of bed. Intuitively, I got to the edge of my bed. I put my good leg on the floor. My whole body was shaking uncontrollably. It was to a point where I couldn't stand there for long. My body resisted my physical efforts, all I could do was hang on with my good arm. Then I crawled back into the bed to rest. My first goal was to stay out of bed for longer periods of time. It was a simple treatment plan. All it required was repetition, patience, courage, discipline and inner strength. I was willing to go to any length to be able to walk again. On three separate occasions throughout the afternoon, I got up, hung on, and shook. I would get so tired that I would have to take short naps.

Ginger came back that evening. She told me she would stay all night with me. This made me feel so much more secure with her there. Feeling tired and secure, I slept throughout the night.

In the morning the nurse brought me breakfast. I didn't feel like eating, so I had a cup of coffee. Ginger needed to go back to her mother's and then to pick my daughter Katie and her husband John from the airport. After Ginger left, I continued with my exercise of getting up, hanging on, and shaking. In the beginning, I was angry at the hospital for being understaffed. I had felt neglected. Now I was viewing this as a positive thing. If the nurses had been in the room, I wouldn't have been able to do my exercise. I was so preoccupied with wanting to walk that time ceased for me.

Ginger, Katie, and John came into the room. I hadn't seen Katie in a couple of years. I had never met her new husband. I was feeling like I had felt with Ginger yesterday, trapped somewhere between worlds. It was such a strange feeling. I was so frustrated because I was unable to communicate with them. Two days had passed, yet no one had talked to me about what had happened. I could see Ginger and Katie were scared and confused. I kept wondering if this was all a dream. I was hoping to wake up and find that I was okay. We didn't know what to do, so we just looked at each other dumbfounded.

When they left, I got out of bed. "Damn," I couldn't stop shaking. I knew my body had been traumatized. I started to talk to my body as though it were a small child who had hurt himself. I assured him that everything would be all right. As I began crying, I looked down at my right side to make sure it was still there. I felt like half of a person. As I hung onto the side of the bed, all I could do was continue crying. In a sense it felt good, it released some of my stuck energy. I pulled myself back into bed and fell asleep.

After sleeping awhile, I got back out of bed. I tried to move my legs and feet across the floor. I felt as though I was going to tip over, I was still shaking. I had trouble lifting my right leg, so I just slid my foot across the floor, while hanging onto the bed. I moved from the head of the bed to the foot of the bed. I knew that I could move no farther, I had pushed myself to the limit. I felt like a child learning to walk. I knew that this was not a question of strength, I had strong legs. It seemed as though the wires to my electrical system were burnt. So somehow, some way I needed to create new pathways in my brain. While I was talking to my body, I started to call it "little Jimmy." Throughout the night little Jimmy and I continued to sleep, shuffle, shake, and hang on.

On Monday, a doctor came into my room. He smiled a lot. He was talking to me, but I couldn't understand what he was saying. Apparently he was from India. He was having difficulty speaking English. I've noticed that when foreign doctors have trouble with their English that they smile a lot. I became frustrated, then angry. I thought, "son-of-a-bitch," he was telling me what had happened to me and I can't even comprehend what he's saying. I suppose he'll charge me five or six hundred dollars for this lousy five minutes of his time. I still didn't know what had happened to me.

The neurologist came in, the first words he uttered were, "You were lucky!" The words echoed in my head. I didn't feel lucky. My left carotid artery was blocked, causing major brain damage, due to lack of oxygen. As if that wasn't bad enough, my right artery was fifty percent blocked. This scared me. I was thinking about my right artery. I wasn't afraid of death, but I was terrorized by the thought of having another stroke on my right side and living through it. I wanted to ask him if he would clean the right artery. I had the question clear in my mind. When I opened my mouth to talk, profanity came out of my mouth; Ginger and the kids looked surprised because they hadn't heard words like that from me. The Doctor appeared embarrassed for them. He proceeded to explain, he can't talk, but at times profanity will spill out of his mouth. He said "even a little old lady, who had never heard words like these in her whole life, she may have words like these slip out of her mouth." No one knows why. My thoughts and feelings went back to my right artery. I had to block these thoughts from my mind. I didn't want to think about this.

My next visitor was a woman from the hospitals' business office. Before she even opened her mouth I knew what she was about to say. "Your insurance won't pay." In one sense I was joyful because they wouldn't keep me here now. On the other hand, I didn't know how I would be able to pay. I was financially broke, and now I couldn't work. I had a sinking feeling in the pit of my stomach.

Five years earlier, in 1987, I had started my own business, ironically I had called it "The Inner Path." When the business failed, I decided to pay my debt, instead of declaring bankruptcy. I gave myself three years to pay off this debt. I had just sent the last check before we came to Fort Myers. I was finally at zero, I didn't owe anybody anything. This hospital bill put me back in debt. I had no way to earn the five thousand dollars I needed to pay it. More pressure, the morning had been devastating.

My left wrist hurt. I looked down to see where the IV needle was. My whole wrist was swollen and red. I pushed the button to call the nurse. He came in, looked at my wrist and left. He returned to give me a pain pill. I cried, pointing to my wrist, he walked away. Lying there helpless, I felt I had no choice but to take the pill. It eased the physical pain, but not the emotional pain I was feeling. I was down and he had run right over me. After the pill wore off, I was back in pain. I pushed the button again. Once more I was frustrated and angry I had no way to communicate or fight back. The nurse knocked me down again by giving me another pill. I had enough, it was a bad day! I didn't sleep very well because I was in so much physical and emotional pain. Feeling powerless, all I could do was hang on. The next morning when Ginger came, I pointed to my wrist. She went to complain, but it was to no avail. They came to check me out of the hospital. They wheeled me down to the business office and I was presented with the bill. The pressure was on. I remember thinking, "I'll pay, but I can't pay today." All of this made me angry. I wanted to sue the hospital, but I knew I wouldn't. Finally we were out of the hospital and on our way home to Sarasota. Suddenly, I couldn't focus my right eye. I hadn't had a problem with it in the hospital. As soon as we got into traffic, my eye started trying to focus everywhere at once. It was as though the eye was receiving confused electrical focusing signals from my brain. It felt like the lens of a fully automatic camera that was stuck on "go," it moved rapidly in and out, trying to focus but never stopping. I had no control over it. My only relief was to close my eyes.

I began to experience extreme anxiety for the first time—that disquieting feeling of uncertainty and foreboding which disturbs the mind and keeps it in a state of painful uneasiness. It was terrifying.

By the time we arrived home, I was exhausted and had to sleep.

Chapter 3

THE BEGINNING OF THE STRUGGLE

When I woke up around four the next morning, I was able to get out of bed. I hung onto the furniture, by sliding my right foot inch by inch I was able to make it into the living room. I sat down. My eyes were giving me trouble and my anxiety level was high. I used my breathing exercises and closed my eyes, trying to relax. My anxiety level soon dropped. I was tired, so I just sat there. My mind started racing. I was thinking about my money situation. After awhile I realized that I was putting excess stress on myself and I shuffled back to the bed.

The next morning, I sat in the living room in a fog. Ginger, Katie, and my other daughter Tammie were busy organizing a plan, Katie called Home Health Services to get a nurse and a speech therapist. Ginger called a neurologist. She also set up an appointment with Health and Rehabilitative Services (HRS). Andrew, a friend who was also a physical therapist called. He offered his service free. Margaret Buzzelli, my employer, called stating that she would help financially. Katie and Tammie began the process of getting papers that I would be needing for HRS and the Social Security Office. They worked all day processing paperwork. I was grateful to them for helping me to live. My wrist still hurt.

Before the stroke I had been very sensitive, now it seemed I was super-sensitive. Because of this, I didn't want anyone to touch me. The energy in the house was so thick, it was overwhelming. I realized that none of us knew what to do. It appeared that we were all in shock. Katie came into the bedroom. She sat down on the edge of the bed. She looked into my eyes while saying, "You have a choice, you can live in Denver with me, in Wisconsin with Laurie, or in Delaware with Tammie." All I could do was smile. I thought, "Is this a joke?" Then I began to cry. I was frustrated because I couldn't communicate what I had become, the pall that draped my eyes like a veil, the reasons I couldn't find shelter in Denver, Wisconsin, or Delaware. Ginger couldn't deal with the idea of me being taken away. My security felt threatened and this scared me. I knew Laurie and Katie moved around a lot and I didn't need or want that. Tammie was the most stable, but still I didn't want to go anywhere. If I had wanted to go somewhere, I would have rented a room somewhere and gone there to lick my wounds. But animals pay no rent, and I had no money. I laid there crying; I wanted to die. Later Ginger came in to tell me that I could stay with her. I was so grateful, and soon fell asleep.

In the early morning, I got up and shuffled into the living room to sit. Andrew and the speech therapist were not able to start until the next week, so I decided to start without them. Intuitively I knew what to do anyway. It had been my vocation for twenty five years. Basically, I would be my client and my therapist.

I was starting to notice that my brain gave me two messages. In my outer reality, I could see and feel that my whole right side is numb, my ankle doesn't bend, my knee is stiff and my arm won't lift up on its own. In my inner reality the opposite was true. The voice was saying that the outer reality was an illusion.

This was the beginning of the struggle or the civil war that erupted and raged on for two years and nine months. I guess that walking engages my brain in a precise electrical and chemical repertoire, each muscle must come into action at a specific moment. If the sequence is altered even slightly, I can fall down.

I decided to use creative visualization. I closed my eyes, I tried to visualize my right leg, the screen in my brain was black. It was like a TV that was off or broken. Before my stroke, every time I closed my eyes I saw colored films playing and I was able to visualize what I wanted. Apparently my TV was damaged. I used to tell my clients, "If you can't get a picture, just think about what you want." Now I would find out if that is true.

I used my left hand to lift up my right leg, I proceeded to think about my left brain and a connection to my ankle to move my foot up and down. After a while, I could feel the resistance in my brain, then I had to rest. Then I did the same thing with my knee and it was the same experience. Then I tried to walk rather then shuffling. It didn't work, I knew that with time, it would. I began this exercise and decided to do it three times a day.

Ginger got up and we had a cup of coffee. I was feeling sad because, before the stroke, every morning we had coffee, breakfast talks and walks through our garden. I desperately wanted to talk with her like we did before. She fixed breakfast and as we ate, I noticed that some way we were communicating with our eyes. I opened my mouth and began to speak, "I wye—veal—;" she seemed to get my message. What I said was "I Love You".

Later I was sitting in a chair and I was trying to write my name. I couldn't write it but I thought that the reason was that I couldn't use my right hand. I put the pencil in my left hand but I still couldn't write it. I realized that I couldn't spell, write and I didn't even remember my kids names. Ginger was sitting there watching me and intuitively she printed each name on the paper including Lucy, my miniature daschund. This was the beginning of my writing exercises. I practiced using both hands.

After lunch, I was exhausted, so I slept. Later I continued doing my exercises.

That evening I checked my blood pressure, it was 90/40. Ginger checked it and finally Katie checked it. It had averaged 91/40. Everyone panicked except me. They said we were going to the emergency room at the hospital. I shook my head no. I hung unto the bed not wanting to let go. They called Andrew, the physical therapist. They talked, leaving me alone. I just wanted to die, maybe it was time. I went to sleep. When I woke up, I thought, "Maybe God doesn't want me either." Maybe my mother and the Church were right, I was going to Hell. I went back to sleep. When I woke again it was four in the morning. I was still here, angry that I didn't die in my sleep. I thought all my problems would be over, if only I would die. That's when it became clear. God must have a plan for me.

Today I had to go to the neurologist. Without thinking about it, I automatically decided to shave like I have for thirty-eight years.

I made my way to the bathroom on the other side of the house. On the trip, I had to sit down to rest. I imagined myself as a little child learning to walk, hanging onto objects as I went. It seemed as if it took forever to get there. When I got there, I got up against the sink and braced my body against the counter, then shifted my weight onto my left leg. I used my left hand to get my shaving gear to the sink. I turned on the hot water, automatically I put my right hand into the hot water and burned myself. I put my shaving cream on my face using my left hand, then put the razor in my right hand and took my left hand grabbing my right wrist, using the left hand to guide it. It worked, except that I was shaking and cut myself numerous times. Then I took toilet paper to put on the cuts. As I was looking in the mirror I had to laugh. At that moment, Ginger came in and smiled. Ginger drove me to the neurologist's office. When I got into the car, I put my left leg into the car forgetting the right leg, I slammed the door on my leg. I felt that! as tears rolled down my cheeks.

When we arrived, I shuffled, dragging my leg to the office. They gave me forms to fill out. I couldn't write so Ginger filled them out for me. The neurologist told us that my left carotid artery was completely clogged. The right carotid artery was fifty percent blocked, coupled with high blood pressure, which prevented the flow of blood to my brain.

I was concerned about my right artery. I couldn't express in words the questions I needed answered. It was so frustrating for me because I had to play charades to get my questions out. I always hated charades, but Ginger was good at this game, so she interpreted my questions for the doctor.

If my right artery became seventy five percent blocked, they would perform surgery. The doctor was concerned about cleaning the artery for fear that I might have another stroke or that it would cause my death. This concerned me too. He said I would need to have a MRI done and also wanted me to have an ultrasound done twice this year, then once every year after that. He wanted to monitor the right artery to make sure that it didn't become more clogged. I didn't have a doctor so he referred me to one in the same complex.

Once again I began worrying about money. I had two hundred dollars left to my name. The neurologists bill came to one hundred eighty five dollars, leaving me with fifteen. I was terrified. I knew I needed the MRI and ultrasound, but I had no money to pay for them. I didn't know how I could possibly pay for these tests and it totally overwhelmed me. I began to deal with my anxiety by using breathing exercises I had learned over the years. After leaving the neurologist's office, we went across the complex to see the other doctor. He examined me and was asking questions. He asked if the blood pressure medicine was affecting my sex performance. My mind reacted in a split second and I felt guilty. I thought that the question was a trick to see if I was having sex, so he could tell me that it's not okay in my condition. He encouraged me to have sex, and I felt relieved. Then we drove to have the ultrasound done. They asked me if I had insurance. Ginger replied, he doesn't know if he has any insurance, it somehow had gotten messed up. The owner and CEO at Anabasis were in the process of straightening it out. The woman at the desk wanted to know how I would pay for the test if my insurance didn't get straightened out. I looked at Ginger. She was honest and stated that he doesn't know. Ginger asked her how much the test would cost. The woman said "Five hundred dollars." Ginger looked at me, I put three fingers up and Ginger told her I would pay in three months. I didn't know how, but I needed to get this test done.

The test itself was an interesting experience. I was able to see the screen while she did the ultrasound. She showed me the blockages in my arteries. She told me my body was producing plaque. She also said it might be an inherited trait. I remembered that my father had a blockage, which he found out about when he was in a car accident. He never did anything about it.

After this test we went to the hospital for my MRI. This time we didn't even ask how much it was going to cost. I'd have to deal with that later. They put me in a tube, I had my eyes open and became very claustrophobic. I closed my eyes, visualizing an open field with beautiful flowers. I tried to keep my breath circular, breath in, breathe out, God in, and back to God. I couldn't focus long on my field of flowers, so I focused on my breathing. Because my attention was focused on my breathing, I lost all track of time. The test felt like it was over in just a matter of minutes, although in reality it had been forty-five minutes. The bill was $1000.00 so I just gave them my insurance card. This had been a long exhausting day. We went home and I slept.

I woke from my nap in time for dinner. I shuffled into the dining room. As I sat there watching Ginger, memories of us cooking together came up and I laughed. She has a cute way that she stands that I adore. I remembered that we had tickets for the theater that Ginger purchased before my stroke. I got her attention and smiled. I tried to say theater and it came out like "ha-te-a." Then I tried again, "ta-tatick," she looked at me and said "Tickets, theater," and smiled. For a moment we were excited to go, then Ginger stated that maybe we shouldn't. I reacted like a little boy that his mother had said no to. I wanted to go, again part of me told me that I was okay. I uttered the following, "I-wa-go;" she threw a sweet smile at me, which made me laugh. Maybe next month.

After dinner, I sat and exercised my ankle and knee. Through the weekend, I was obsessed with my exercising, visualizing and trying to write the names on the list that Ginger made up. I practiced using both hands and would try to say the names out loud. Each morning at 5 A.M., I would begin to exercise. After a while it became a discipline.

The next week, Andrew, my physical therapist, came to help me with my walking exercises. The work that I was already doing was what he wanted me to do. He added some balancing exercises, that consisted of having me stand in front of the kitchen counter and hang on, then I would lift one leg up and try to let go and balance, then I would switch legs. I added this exercise to my program in my head.

As usual, the nurse came every morning to check my blood pressure. The speech therapist came to set up a program. She told me that she would see me three days a week. As I tried to put my feelings into words a jumbled stream of verbal double talk spewed from my lips. Little did I know at this time how involved communication really was. I was told I had something called aphasia, but no one had explained what it was. If I had known, I would have given up right then. But I didn't give up, I added another aspect to my treatment plan. She gave me sheets of single words to practice saying out loud. I decided to practice one hour a day, seven days a week. I couldn't remember or say her name. I tried the word, "Teach" and found that after a while I could say it.

Teach had brought a tongue depressor with her. When I would try to get a word out and it wouldn't come, she would stick that tongue depressor in my mouth, as if to force the word out of my mouth. I don't think she understood that I had the word in my head, but my brain wouldn't let the word come out. No matter how many times she put that depressor in my mouth, she couldn't force that word from my brain to my lips. That damn stick was making me angry. I looked right at her and thought, "If you put that stick in my mouth one more time,

I'm going to stick it up your ass!" She must have gotten my message telepathically, because she never brought that stick back again. Now we were able to become friends. After Teach left, I had lunch, and then it was off to HRS for my one o'clock appointment.

Once at HRS, we had to wait forty-five minutes to see my counselor. We were finally let into her office and she went over all of my paperwork. She knew from the paperwork that I had suffered a stroke, but apparently she didn't understand how strokes can affect people. I tried to answer her questions, but I couldn't, so Ginger talked for me. I wanted to ask her how many food stamps I would be getting. Automatically I started to ask. Even though I couldn't talk, my mouth opened and profanity poured through my lips. It was like my experience in the hospital. She jumped out of her chair, looked me in the eye and said, "No one uses those words in my office. If you are going to use those words in my office get out!" I felt total shame and embarrassment as I began to cry. I was worried they wouldn't give me any food stamps because of an outburst that I had no control over. I felt like a small child who had been scolded. However my crying seemed to calm her down. She approved my request for food stamps. I would be getting one hundred eleven dollars a month. I went with my little blue card to stand in a line. I couldn't stand up any longer, so Ginger went and got a supervisor who allowed her to go to the front of the line, while I sat down. I was feeling shame as I was sitting there. I attacked myself with thoughts of, "Look at yourself! You're worthless!" My pride of being able to take care of myself was crushed. I moved those thoughts out of the way. Ginger received my food stamps and we were on our way to the grocery store.

I needed to eat a low-fat diet. I also needed to eat more fruits, along with vegetables and drink more juices. Because of this, I was trying to pick out low fat, low salt foods. This was when I discovered that I couldn't read the labels. Now I realized that even though I could see the word, my mind didn't comprehend it. I found that sometimes I couldn't see the word at all. Ginger read the labels to me. Sometimes what she said wouldn't register in my brain, so she ended up picking out my food for me.

My next discovery was that I can't buy a healthy diet on one hundred eleven dollars a month. Health is very expensive. It's kind of sad.

When we got to the register my food stamps didn't cover my purchases. Ginger paid the difference. I was tired, it had been another long, frustrating day. We went home and I went to sleep.

The next day while I did my exercises, Katie and Tammie went to the Social Security Office to start the process of getting my Social Security Disability. It was their understanding, that while we were waiting for my disability payments to be approved, I would be eligible to receive SSI payments. I did receive an SSI payment, but not until six months later, when I received my first disability payment. They found that I wouldn't get any Medicare for two years after the disability. This concerned me, because if I had to go to the hospital again I don't know what I would do.

That afternoon I practiced reading the words on my sheets. I struggled with the words. After a while I started feeling sorry for myself. No one understood what I was going through. Just then Ginger's dog Lucy jumped in my lap. I couldn't say her name, so I called her (WENR) Wiener. To this day I still call her Wiener. She looked at me and I knew she understood. She comforted me in a way that no human had been able to. She somehow helped me get through my self pity.

The next day we had to go to Fort Myers. Both the HRS and Social Security Office required a copy of my hospital records. Katie had called two weeks prior to this and requested the records be sent. They never came, so we had to go to Fort Myers to get them. I was so angry, it seemed that no one gave a damn about me. I had to go all the way down there because the hospital required my signature before they would release my records. As we drove into Fort Myers, we stopped to have some lunch. The restaurant we stopped at was extremely busy. The three of us didn't even think about my condition, as I shuffled and hung on to Ginger and Katie. The noises made my brain feel as though it were short circuiting. I began to experience panic. We looked at each other, it was like we were thinking the same thoughts. I had to get out of there. I shuffled back to the car, trying to calm myself down. We continued on our way to the hospital. As we approached the hospital I felt my whole body react to its cold omnipresent atmosphere. It was as if every cell in my body recalled the trauma I had suffered here. My anxiety went higher and higher with each step we took towards the business office. I thought I was going to have another stroke. We entered the office. I couldn't sign my name so I scribbled something. I thought, "This is so ridiculous, I had to come all the way down here to scribble on a piece of paper." They gave me my file and we were on our way back to Sarasota. By the time we reached home I was completely worn out, I needed to sleep.

The next morning I did my usual exercises, I also did some work with the speech therapist. This was a frustrating task for me. I had clear images in my mind, but when I tried to get the words from my mind to my mouth, they wouldn't come. I tried to look up the word aphasia in the dictionary. I discovered that I lost my A-B-C's—Where did they go? My brain drew a blank as I struggled to find them. After struggling for a half hour, I found the word. When I tried to read the meaning, I couldn't comprehend what I just read so I read it over and over. I got one word, "speechless." I knew that before I did all that work! So, at that time, I still didn't know the dynamics of that word. As I went along, I discovered that I couldn't recognize or recall numbers or dates, I couldn't add, subtract, or divide. When I made coffee, I would count, 1-5-3-7-10. Consequently my coffee was usually strong. It took forever to read the directions just to get a simple frozen dinner cooked.

I was finally realizing just how much damage my brain had suffered. Before the stroke I never thought about my brain or how it functioned. Now that I didn't have full use of it, I was beginning to understand how much I really need it just to survive in this world. This scared me. I didn't know if I would get any better.

It's like the electrical system in your house. If a hurricane knocks out the power and everything that you depend on for your survival is gone, how do you feel? The difference with your house is someone can fix the damage and your power will be restored. With brain damage, no one can fix it. I had to block my thoughts on this, or else I would shoot myself.

It was time for Katie and Tammie to leave. There we were, sitting there all alone, Ginger was sitting on the couch, me in a chair that faced her. The house was in total silence that was deafening. Our eyes were hooked together as though we were one. No words were spoken, it was as though our communication link was telepathic. It seems that both of us were thinking the same thing, "Now what do we do. We are all alone." We sat there for a moment in the stillness and oneness with no fear, just peace with tears running down our cheeks. Just a moment before the storm.

My employer Peg Buzzelli and her daughter came to visit. Ginger talked and interpreted my communication. At one point Peg stated to me, "You need to write a book." I looked at Ginger shaking my head. Ginger told her that I can't write. Peg stated, type it. I thought that maybe I could. When they left, I went to the typewriter and discovered that I couldn't type. The days and weeks progressed. I continued with my exercises, but I was still having trouble with my balance and my walking. I always felt like I was going to tip over. There were times when I actually did tip over. Then I remembered a stick that I had put in my closet. It had a roach clip on one end and a painted florescent ball on the other. One of my clients had given it to me. I remembered that it had something to do with focusing, so I clipped it to the front of my hat. Then I went out to the shuffleboard court. I focused on the ball. It gave me a sense of balance, as I tried to walk. I tried it at night in the dark and it worked just as well. I called it my walking stick. My ankle and knee were beginning to work. They would try to resist walking and would get tight, but I pushed them. I used my walking stick and would walk forward from one end of the shuffleboard court to the other, then I would walk backwards to where I started. As long as I focused on the ball, I could walk a straight line. Since I was getting up at five in the morning, I could do my walking exercises even though the sun wasn't up. I felt more secure when I used my walking stick. I was so excited about how well my walking stick was working for me that I thought I could market it for people who had trouble walking. When I discussed this idea with my physical therapist, he dismissed the idea. I thought, "To hell with you! What do you know? You seem to think I have a problem with my muscles." In fact it wasn't my muscles at all, my brain wasn't sending the right messages to my body.

I finally reached the point in my treatment where I was ready to move from the shuffleboard court to the street. I wanted to see how far and how fast I could walk in one hour. Ginger and I measured the route for one mile. Trying to walk that mile in one hour would be my first goal. I left the driveway, moving at a pretty good pace. However after a short distance my body tightened up as if it didn't want to walk any farther. The resistance in the right side of my body was tremendous. I had to sit down.

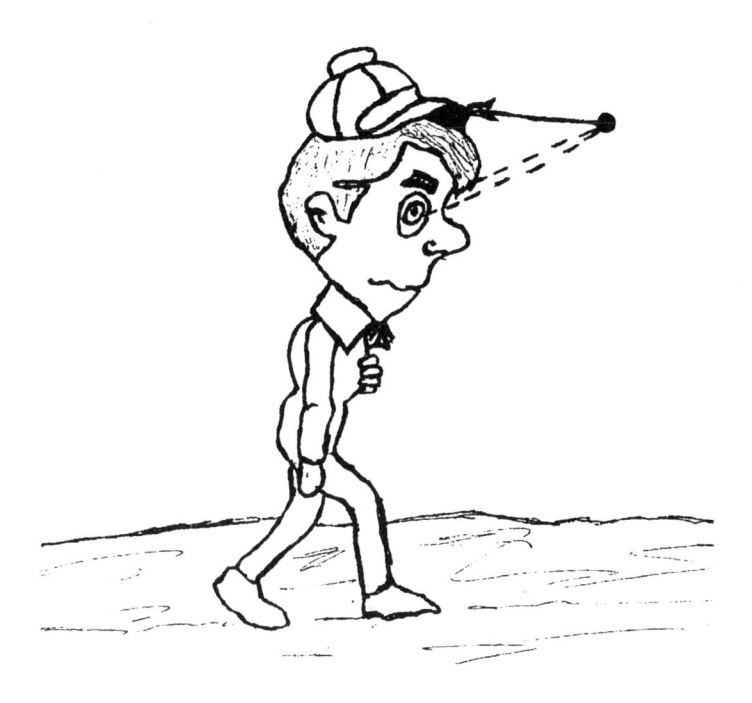

Because of my past experience, I decided to use my breath work and visualization on my next walk. The following day I left the driveway visualizing I was a plane taxiing down the runway. At the same time I was breathing systematically from my diaphragm. This worked well for me, but because of the damage done to my brain, I couldn't concentrate for any period of time. Even though I'd lose my concentration, the diaphragmatic breathing brought more oxygen into my bloodstream, while at the same time keeping my body more relaxed. Before my stroke I had helped many of my clients get on top of their addictions by teaching breath work. I had set up my business, "The Inner Path," to teach people the breath work techniques that I had learned over the years. My body also responded favorably to my visualization. Because I was focusing on being a plane, my attention was drawn away from my right side, making my body less tense. This enabled me to walk farther than I had yesterday.

When I got home I had my breakfast. This consisted of a variety of fruit, toast, orange juice, and grapefruit juice, which I squeezed myself.

Then I read out loud for an hour. I tired easily, so at eleven o'clock I would sleep. When I woke up I'd have my lunch consisting of vegetables, salad, V8 juice, and milk.

In the afternoon I would practice reading words out loud. My right eye continued giving me trouble, making me so dizzy I'd have to sit down and close my eyes. I felt as though I were spinning out of control. So along with my diaphragmatic breathing I tried eye exercises.

Then I would spend time with Wiener, she could always make me feel good. She was my psychotherapist when I was getting into self-pity.

I'd be tired again so I'd go to sleep for a while.

After waking up I'd watch CNN news. Then I'd have dinner consisting of vegetables and rice, or a comparable low fat meal, cleaning up the kitchen after I was finished. Then Ginger and I would go for a swim at the beach. I was told that I shouldn't be swimming in the gulf. It angered me. First of all, when people tell me that I can't, then I will. Secondly, I hate it when people think that they are in charge of my body and my life. I have always felt very comfortable in the water, and I believe that salt water has healing properties. I incorporated swimming as part of my treatment plan. Before my stroke, Ginger and I went to the beach in the evening, I got two benefits, swimming and gorgeous sunsets.

My body felt better while I was swimming and floating. I understand why people were trying to dissuade me, because they assumed that I was weak from my stroke, but I wasn't. My muscles were strong, because I got up right away in the hospital so that my muscles wouldn't become weak.

My routine was pretty much set. Seven days each week I'd wake up and start over, continually trying to balance all the aspects of my life. In the front of my mind there was always a vision of my being able to become balanced in my physical, emotional, mental, social, and spiritual levels. My ultimate goal was to at least become as good as I was before the stroke and possibly better.

One morning my right leg was giving me trouble. Before I left for my walk, I tried to loosen it up with some yoga exercises. I went out the driveway trying to visualize myself as a plane taxiing down the runway. I couldn't concentrate, my leg was getting tighter. I slowed down trying to concentrate on my breathing. When I got my breathing into a rhythmic pattern, I continued on. After a short distance my leg became even tighter. It felt painful, even though it was numb. I couldn't understand this. I usually experienced this tightness at the beginning of a walk, but it usually loosened up during the walk. It was as if my body was resisting this exercise, almost as though it wanted to stay home and sit on the lanai not doing anything.

When I was about a mile away from home, my leg refused to carry me any farther. I fell over into the grass. As I lay there, I started talking with my body. "Okay little Jimmy, we're a mile away from home and no one knows where we are." I could have sworn that he answered me, saying, "I don't want to walk anymore." So I said, "Okay we'll just lay here. You're in charge, I can't get up without you." I just lay there breathing. My dialogue with little Jimmy continued. Finally little Jimmy grudgingly gave in. I was able to get off the ground, I started toward home. Little Jimmy gave me trouble all the way home. I continued with my breathing exercises, and was able to make it home, then I took a nap.

Finally, I came to the point where I made the decision that I had to drive. I no longer wanted to be dependent on Ginger or anyone else to drive me to my appointments.

I was concerned about the welfare of others, and aware that I would be criticized for attempting to drive, but my increasing need for independence and my hunger to be self-sufficient dictated my decision. My right eye was improving and I had perfectly clear vision in my left one. My reflexes were good.

I began driving the car forward and backward in the driveway. I practiced this for a few days until I was confident enough to drive around the block. My oldest daughter, Laurie, who had come for a two week visit, acted as my copilot. Her sister Katie yelled at her because she didn't think I should drive and Laurie told her "You know Dad, he is so determined to get well, so it would be better to help him."

Every day we drove to the village and back. Even though others discouraged me from driving, I chose to focus on this additional phase of my recovery. I made it to the bridge that would take me to the mainland. I was afraid to cross over the first time and so I pulled into a little park by the bridge to rest. I practiced my breathing exercises until I was calm, then drove myself home. I had always driven defensively, and I thought that now I would be even more defensive and I vowed always to stop and rest if I felt any stress or fear.

I resigned myself to just driving around Siesta Key for a while. Soon the Key seemed to grow smaller and smaller and I wanted to venture farther. I needed to overcome any fear of driving to the mainland because that was where my doctor and shopping were.

Finally, I made it over the bridge, anxiety and all! As my confidence and skill incresed, my driving gave me a new found freedom and ability to seek wellness.

One day while I was out doing errands I stopped at the grocery store. This was where I discovered that I didn't know how to figure my money. I could see the numbers on the bills, but I couldn't comprehend what it was worth. I looked at the amount on the register and didn't know how much to give the cashier. I asked the woman behind me for help, but because of my garbled speech she didn't understand me. I think I frightened her because she moved to another register. I pushed my money towards the cashier. She pushed it back. I felt retarded and started to cry. I finally got the attention of another woman and pleaded "Lehp Me!" I pointed to the total on the register, she understood and counted out my money for me. The hopelessness I felt was overwhelming. I left the store the tears still glistening in my eyes.

Numerous clients and friends came to see me. Because I physically looked good, it was only when I opened my mouth that they would realize that I wasn't the same. It must have scared them because they never came back after the first visit.

As I started going out more on a social level, I found people accepting me because of my physical appearance, but once again when I opened my mouth I felt socially unacceptable. Ginger and I continued going to the theater, to parties, and to dinners. I tried not to talk, my anxiety was high, so I would concentrate on my breathing.

Everyday I was continually having to work at keeping my positive attitude. It was hard work. You've heard the phrase, "One day at a time," well most days I had to take it one hour at a time. Other days I'd have to take it one breath at a time.

I tried to live each day to its fullest, because I never knew if it would be my last.

After working very hard to get back to the way I was before the stroke, Ginger and I decided to take a little trip for some relaxation. We didn't realize that we were both still in shock from the trauma. We both thought that I was as good as new. Ginger had found a deal on some round trip airline tickets, that were ninety dollars apiece. I didn't have any money so she decided for my birthday, she would take me on a trip to Montana. I had lived there before I moved to Sarasota. She had never been there. Ginger told the nurse and speech therapist. They just looked at us in disbelief. The nurse freaked out and stated, don't tell me, don't tell me, don't tell me or I'll have to report it. I really felt a deep sense that I had to go, so it wouldn't have made any difference who disagreed with me, I was going.

This trip made me aware that when there was a lot of noise and talking, my brain would shut down. My brain was like a fuse box with wires hanging down. When the wires would hit against each other, they would go "zzzzzz, zzzzzz, ZAP," until I blew a fuse. Every time I would try to comprehend everything going on around me, I would blow a fuse. The lights in my mind would go out and I was left in the dark.

When we arrived in Montana we rented a car. Ginger had never driven in the mountains, so I drove. I was comfortable driving, because of my past experience of driving in the mountains, my intuition took over. We went north toward Big Fork, taking the east road around Flat Head Lake, a huge deep glacier lake, that doesn't freeze in the winter. As we drove through the cherry orchards on the banks of the lake, it took me back to the past springtimes. I could smell the sweet cherry blossoms and taste the ripened cherries. I tried to share my experience with Ginger and it seemed that she was in tune with me. After some time on the road, I noticed feelings of serenity. My electrical system seemed calm. I was feeling cool breezes in the air and I could feel the winter approaching. We decided to stay in Big Fork, a small town, nestled in the foothills of the mountains, surrounded by Federal forests, and sitting at the mouth of Flat Head River. The scenery is breathtaking. I'd compare it to the scenery in the movie "The River Runs Through It." Big Fork could be described as an artist community.

In the morning, we drove to Kalispell where I used to live, then to Whitefish and went up in the ski lifts to a restaurant for lunch. The restaurant has a view of the entire Flat Head Valley. As we were going down the slopes, a bear was running beneath us, Ginger got excited and I had to laugh, she was squealing like a little kid. We got off on the bottom and walked to the car.

We continued on heading toward Glacier. When we arrived at Glacier Park, it was getting colder. My right side was hurting from the cold. We rented a cabin on McDonald Lake. I turned the heat on to get my body settled down and took my blood pressure reading. It was good. Later we went to dinner. Ginger had been ordering for me and she told me to see if I could order for myself. I tried, a couple of words came out, cgf-s-ds and at the same time I was pointing to the menu. I felt embarrassed, but it passed. After dinner we stood on the shore of the mountain lake at sundown. We looked across the rippling, limpid lake, past the dark forest, into the heart of a flaming fading sky, isolated clouds were floating by and the pines were chanting like the sea. God seemed very near to me, here in the forest, I felt a oneness with nature. Then a full moon came into view, a silvery beauty shimmering with points of light like diamonds. The wind danced through Ginger's hair and it took me back to when we first met. It was a night like this, on Turtle Beach. As we sat there, the night clouds came to blanket the peaks of the mountains.

The next day we went higher into the mountains to explore several hiking trails. My mind seemed clear. I believed that I was running up and down the trail. Ginger told me that I could hardly drag my leg down the trail, however I was able to go quite a distance.

It was a good exercise. The terrain helped with my balance, however my ankle and knee would resist at times.

Being in the park brought back memories. I came here in the summer seasons on weekends, to commune with nature. It was so peaceful, serene, and clean. I didn't want to leave. I was thinking, why did I leave this to go live in the swamp, but then I thought I felt the same peacefulness and serenity in the swamp. We were ready to go higher into the mountains. I had Ginger drive, so I could give her some pointers in mountain driving, in case that something would happen to me. I gave her a very simple crash course: 1. Shift down when your going down in order to utilize the engine power instead of the brakes. If your going too fast for the curves, brake, shift down again, then just go up and down using the transmission rather than the brakes. 2. Change your thinking, the curves are the same whether you are on flat roads or up and down roads. With that course, she did great.

We went higher, then stopped to check the map of the different hiking trails. We found one that would take us into a beautiful lake.

It was a beautiful fall day, the temperature was in the high 60s. The sun was bright, radiating life to all things in the forest, birds were singing and the wind crooned through the trees. The landscape seemed thoughtful, reflective, a little wistful. We hiked up and down, Ginger in the front, me dragging my behind. We proceeded toward the lake and I sat on a rock on its shore in awe. Ginger walked farther down its shore and turned to face the water. The lake looked like a huge jewel set into the mountain. As the sun gleamed and sparkled on its surface, it reflected light on Ginger's face. It was awesome. I knew my hungry heart needed this kind of beauty. There she was, the goddess of nature. I always felt that Ginger was a nature goddess trying to be a city girl, causing her conflict within.

We hiked back to the car and drove higher, on the road that they call "The Road To The Sun." We climbed higher and higher reaching toward the sun, until we could see where we came from. Ginger's driving was excellent; I felt comfortable and I don't trust too many on this road. We climbed and climbed, going past the Wall of Tears. The mountain weeps, it's nature's way to express itself. The energy on the wall was heavy as we passed. It was weeping, sending tears onto the road. It was a sign that the death of winter was upon us. We continued our climb toward the Sun and finally we hit the summit. We hiked on the summit but the air was so thin I had a hard time breathing so we left.

As we were descending, going down the other side, we stopped to view a mountain goat and her baby. They stood there and watched us. Their fur appeared heavy, ready for the winter blow. Farther down we were confronted with a bear. He was trying to eat his belly full so he could get out of the winter's death. It was interesting to me that Ginger's animal spirit is the bear.

We stopped at St. Mary lake and got a room in the old Lodge. They had only a few rooms left. It was unusual to have so many people this late in the season. We had a wonderful dinner and sat in front of a huge fireplace. I was dead tired and the heat from the fireplace was about to put me to rest.

In the morning I could see the signs that snow was approaching. We took a hike, but to get to the trail we had to take a boat. We brought some rain and snow gear and proceeded to find the trail. We found the trail and it was starting to rain, the white clouds were forming in the west. It appeared that snow was coming. It made me a little uncomfortable. As we hiked the trail, I could hear the little critters moving about, nature was busy for the upcoming winter. We spotted two large moose grazing about ten yards away. We stopped, I remember the stillness. It was so still, we could hear them breathing. We stood there in awe. Later we moved on, toward the lake. Snow had already begun falling by the time we got to the lake, and the scene was breathtaking. My mind went back to summer, where life moved, showing its beauty. The death of winter, with its stillness and peace seemed the same. We hiked back to the boat. When we arrived back at the lodge, we had dinner and then sat watching the fire in the fireplace.

It was still snowing the next morning when we woke up. They had closed the west side of The Road To The Sun, so we had to leave the Lodge. We continued on to St. Mary's. The snow was getting deeper, and the wind was picking up. I was afraid we would be driving into a blizzard. Since Ginger had never driven in the snow, I took over. The wind was blowing the snow so fast we couldn't see the road. I know the road, so I hugged the mountain to my left and prayed that another car wouldn't be there. Once again someone was watching over and guiding us. One slip of the car and we would have been careening down the side of the mountain.

Throughout the trip, I found I wouldn't have been able to function there by myself because of my problem with my speech. I couldn't order food, or pay for it. I couldn't ask for directions. I couldn't even register for the cabin.

The cold affected my right side. It felt like a toothache. It became so sensitive that I couldn't even touch it. All of this was very frustrating for me. I had some anxiety, thinking, "What if I have another stroke?" As I became more aware of the things I couldn't do, I realized these were new fears I hadn't experienced before.

When this wonderful trip finally ended, I was feeling sadness. On the flight home, I couldn't express my true feelings and experiences to Ginger. I felt isolated and trapped between worlds. I felt so much love toward her that I thought I would burst. I felt a sacred communion with her and nature and I couldn't express it. I felt an energy that gave me strength to get through what I was about to experience.

After arriving home, I got back to my routine. I still had my membership at the YMCA so I added that to my exercise program. Now that I could drive to the mainland, I started going over and using the weight machines. People were telling me I shouldn't be doing that type of exercising. But it made me feel better. My body was in good shape; physically I looked good, so I ignored everyone and continued my exercise. By using the machines at the YMCA I was able to lower my blood pressure some. By doing my breathing exercises with my workouts, I was getting more oxygen into my blood stream. I knew that oxygen was just as important to the vitality of every cell in my body as was the food I ate to fuel it.

Around the fifth month of my disability, Home Health Services decided I wouldn't get any better. I sensed this even though they didn't talk to me about it. I had improvement in my walking and my speech, but I had yet to discover all the dynamics of aphasia. Emotionally and mentally I was a mess and I knew I wasn't happy with the quality of my life at this time.

A social worker was sent to the house and he referred me to Vocational Rehabilitative Services. I tried to find out why they were referring me there. He wouldn't be honest with me. This only reinforced the feeling that I wasn't going to get any better. They wanted to train me to sit in one of the Goodwill collection trailers.

At this point Social Security was still dragging their feet on making a decision on my case, even though they knew I was disabled. They forced me to go to Vocational Rehabilitative Services. I felt my survival was being threatened, which in turn triggered all kinds of fear and anxiety. This only intensified all the fear and anxiety I had been feeling the last four months. I didn't understand their views. I was still in shock from the initial trauma. I wasn't feeling stable in any area of my life. I went to my appointment with the Vocational Rehabilitative Services. As I sat there listening to the counselor, I thought, "These people don't understand." I tried to explain to her that even though I looked good physically, my right side was numb and I was afraid I would hurt myself lifting boxes into the Goodwill trailer. She just smiled at me. I've noticed that when people don't understand, they smile a lot. I was so frustrated by not being able to express my concerns and feelings, that I slumped down in the chair and cried. My eye was going every which way but loose. At this point I felt I shouldn't drive home. The stress, my money situation, everything I had been going through these past months seemed to cave in on top of me. I couldn't catch my breath. I thought I was going to have another stroke. At this point the counselor said she would check with me in a few months.

It seemed as though I would just catch my breath and then my world would fall down around me. There was a letter from Social Security waiting for me when I got home. They ordered me to be seen by their psychologist. The appointment was set for the following month. I felt deflated, then I noticed the newspaper on the coffee table with a list of stroke support groups in Sarasota. In the list were two stroke survivor groups. I called the first number. I was having trouble talking with the lady, because of my aphasia. Somehow I got across to her that I was the victim of a stroke. She started to give me a telephone number. I told her to say one number at a time, slowly. She said, "Okay." She finished saying the number before I could even write one number. I told her, "One number at a time." She rattled the number off again. I was so frustrated, I hung up. This had been a bad day, but I decided to try the other group. It was a repeat of what had just happened. I hung up again.

Finally I found another support group, but when I went to the meeting no one was there. I thought, "Three strikes and you're out!"

I had an appointment with the neurologist and he had gotten my second ultrasound test back. He told me that I had a good flow of blood and oxygen to my brain and the artery was the same. It felt good to hear that, but I sensed that the medical end of my treatment was finished. I guess I had been fixed. I didn't feel fixed.

The day after Thanksgiving I became ill with the flu. I hadn't been sick for twenty-five years. I was so sick, I thought I was going to die, I actually hoped I would. It felt as though my whole being was going through a threshing machine, separating the chaff from the grain.

Through the previous five months my progress was good. I was walking and my speech had improved. The flu put me back in bed. I regressed back to the point where I had started in Fort Myers. In a sense this was worse! I couldn't lift my head off my pillow. I tried to get out of bed, but I couldn't. I was afraid I would never get up again. It was as if I couldn't struggle any more. I was angry and had no way to vent my anger. I was stuck with it. I was completely dependent on another human being, just like a new born child. I thought if this is the rock bottom, at least there's only one way to go, and that was up. At this point in time, I didn't realize that this was not the bottom.

The days progressed into weeks. I lay helpless. It took all the strength I could muster to move my head to the edge of the bed, just so I could throw up in a bucket. I could crawl to the bathroom and Ginger was able to lift me up. I couldn't eat and was becoming weaker. I knew I had to eat, but I had to settle for broth. I lost all track of time, becoming delirious at times. I would get up only to fall back down. As time went on I was able to get myself out of bed, shake, and hang on. My head felt like it was going to burst. Each day I would get up and do what I did in the hospital, get out of bed, shake, and hang on.

I woke one morning, it was still dark and I was still delirious. I was able to get out of bed, but I didn't know where I was going. I was in a fog as I shuffled out of the bedroom, not aware that Ginger was following me. In the dining room was a six foot glass table. As I shuffled past the table I passed out. As I fell under the table, the glass top started to fall on me. Ginger grabbed the glass, holding onto it while at the same time pulling me out from under the table. She put me back into bed and I slept. When I woke the next morning, I felt the whole episode had been a dream.

As time passed I began to get better. Soon I emerged from my sickness. Now I was slowly able to get back into my exercises. Because I had been sick for over a month, I had lost all the benefits I had gained after the stroke. I had regressed back to the point where I was when I had the stroke. I had to start over from the very beginning. Within a few weeks of hard work I was able to get my speech and walking back to where it had been before I contracted the flu. I realized now that my immune system was not up to par.

Before my stroke, I seldom got sick or had any allergies and few colds. Now it seemed as if every bug, germ, dust and pollen were attacking. I started experiencing colds, allergy symptoms, sneezing, coughing and my sinuses went wild. It didn't matter if I was walking sitting or lying down, I couldn't breath. I tried numerous cold and allergy medicines, all to no avail. Then I tried Afrin Nasal Spray. I knew it was a bad thing for me to use, but to get any relief so I could breath. As time marched on, I had only used it when I went to bed, then I was using it twice a day. Within a year I was sniffing it every hour, it was like cocaine, except I didn't get off on it.

Chapter 4

JOURNEY TO HELL

Depression hit me, immense darkness began. A profusion of darkness which came creeping in, swallowed me up. The blackest hours of my present existence were about to begin. I remembered from past lessons in my recovery from my alcoholism and working with clients that depression is a normal and basically healthy phenomenon. It signals that a major change is happening. The old must be given up in order to allow the new to come in. The giving-up process often begins with a period of intense crisis, chaos, conflict and darkness. It is an integral part of the process of mental and spiritual growth. Even though I knew this through experience, my whole being reacted so quickly that I struggled against being pulled downward. I used my breathing exercises to try and lift this heaviness I was feeling. As I descended into the darkness, I was filled with suffering and uncertainty. Each day it was pulling me further down into the blackness. I felt that I was torn in different directions, physically, emotionally, and mentally. I felt as though I was moving through a perilous, mysterious realm called the void. It was so heavy, the weight of it shown in my physical body. I couldn't stand up straight. Ginger commented on this and even physically tried to push my body up. Also I was having trouble with my breathing. Emotionally I was numb, while mentally I shut myself off from the outer world automatically. I was spiraling downward not knowing if I would ever stop my descent. I was feeling terror in my heart. The darkness thickened as I descended into a greasy cesspool and was totally engulfed in it, yet I was aware of my outer world. I could see and sense that Ginger was getting spooked, but I couldn't do anything about it.

Ginger sat me down and said, "The sparkle in your eyes is gone." I could see and sense her fear and I felt so powerless, I began to cry. I couldn't explain and express what was happening to me. She wanted to know if I still loved her. I tried to explain, that I felt dead inside and I had no feelings for anything. I couldn't express in a way that would help her understand. I sensed that she felt that I didn't love her. I had a sick, sinking feeling that our relationship was strained to the point of breaking, I just sat there hunched over.

It seemed that every day I went down deeper and deeper, trying to hang on. After a while, I couldn't hang on any more. As I was letting go, something seemed to slow my descent. I felt a stillness and a peace envelop me in perfect gentleness, dropping me as gently as snowflakes falling weightless, rocking me softly as a feather.

The struggle was over and I was at peace. I wanted to stay right where I was. I didn't understand what was happening to me. Is this what the church called "purgatory"? I didn't know if this was a dream or if there actually was a voice telling me, "This is the other side of God." Slowly I was able to climb out of the inky darkness into the gray. I got out of my depression around Christmas, but my mood wasn't all that great. I still needed to deal with my immune system, including my sinus problem, eye, speech and anxieties.

I began to take vitamins to help me with my immune system. I started using a powdered C, a multi B-complex, and a multi-vitamin. Apparently, there is a man in the sky that tells all the vitamin factories your name and address. I began to get vitamin catalogs in the mail. I hung on, resisting buying some of the miracle pills. I bought a book and in it was a section on vitamins that helped the brain, so I started to order them. In awhile, I had a big bag of vitamins that I took with me wherever I went. I was embarrassed popping pills. One day Ginger and a friend went to lunch. The friend had a big bag of vitamins and she told Ginger that she was embarrassed and wanted to come to the house to pop her pills. Ginger laughed and told her that Jim has a big bag too, he'll love it. She came over and we popped pills together. I began to look at my obsession with vitamins and realized that taken in such excess, they might even be toxic to my system. I decided to return to my original vitamin dosage.

It was New Years Eve. We went to a house party at some friends, and I was still down. I tried to get myself up, but wasn't successful. I was glad that Ginger had a good time. A week later we had another party and I felt a little better. I tried talking with people and Ginger was talking with this guy. After we left Ginger stated that he told her, "Get rid of that old fart," meaning me. It angered me, but I thought, maybe I'm looking like an old fart, I was feeling that way.

The frequency and depth of anxiety episodes were becoming so severe that I had started to think that I would give in and get some Xanax just to take the edge off at the worst times. This was very dangerous for me. I wanted to be very cautious because of the hundreds of people I have helped trying to get off of this drug. But I finally went to the doctor and told him to give me one month's prescription, low dose, and NO REFILLS. The Xanax in low dose did seem to help when the attacks were serious and I was grateful for the relief. I was fearful of becoming dependent on this chemical relief, and remained alert to its dangers. I never tried to refill the prescription.

Chapter 5

SOCIAL SECURITY

I was worried about my Social Security Disability. I still had not received a decision on my case. Ginger had called the office numerous times during this process. They had all the information they needed, yet they were holding up my disability payments. The avalanche of bills I was receiving only made me worry more. I felt helpless, angry and ignored, and not being able to verbally express these emotions was a constant frustration.

We weren't getting any satisfaction, so Ginger wrote to the Congressman Senator, and we pressured the social services agencies in Tallahassee. I felt it was a stalling tactic when they forced me to see a psychologist.

I went to the appointment with the psychologist angry and impatient. Although I couldn't articulate my anxiety and anger, I sensed that he was empathetic and would report my obvious need for help.

Soon I received a letter from Social Security explaining that I was eligible for Disability payments in the reduced amount of only $900 per month. I was very disappointed because they told Katie that I should receive between $1500 and $2000 each month.

Since my daughter Laurie had recently moved nearby in Sarasota, she was able to help me. She took me to the Social Security office. They pulled up my records from their computer. When we looked at the computer printout,we found there were several discrepancies in my earnings. They had one year of income out of the three years that I had spent in the Navy. They had no record for the year I worked for the State of Wisconsin. The income it showed for my ten years at Uniroyal was less than what I was paying to send my three girls through Catholic School. For the two years I was a carpet layer, there was no income listed at all. Twenty-five years out of my forty-three years of working were wrong. My mind couldn't comprehend how this could be.

To correct this, we would have to produce my W2s. We tried to get copies of my W2s, but most businesses had thrown them away after seven years.

If you don't get anything else from this book but one thing, I recommend that you check every three years with Social Security to make sure your earnings are correct. If they're not correct, you'll need your W2s before they will correct them. Always keep your W2s.

Chapter 6

OH NO, NOT THE TRAILER!

It was six months after my stroke when I received another letter from Vocational Rehabilitative Services. They had decided without seeing me that I was well enough to be retrained. I knew I wasn't well enough to work. I had just received my Social Security Disability and I feared they would take it away. I could feel this gnawing in the pit of my stomach. Now they wanted to train me to sit in a trailer. I was so angry, all the literature and information I had read and learned indicated that it took two to three years to recuperate from a major stroke. Now they wanted me to go back to work. I still couldn't speak. I still had trouble with my balance and my right side was still numb.

I went to my appointment. I was angry, I cried, I pleaded, "Not the trailer! I'm not an idiot." Whatever self confidence I had gained in the past months, she took away from me with the pretense of helping me. I thought to myself, I see many young people trying to get training to no avail. Why not spend their money on some young person who needed and wanted their training? Why would they want to retrain me at this point. I needed time to heal and work at getting my speech and motor skills back.

In my mind I was still the same person, with many, many skills. I was aware of everything, but the vehicle of expression from the mind was damaged. The mind and the brain are separate, yet I need to use the brain as a vehicle to expression. My brain sends the message, my mind wants sent. My mind was trapped, my damaged brain could not send the messages.

Apparently the counselor understood. She referred me to a psychologist for testing.

When I went to the appointment with the psychologist, I wasn't informed that it would be all day testing. I tried to explain to her that I needed to have a nap in the afternoon. I would go home at noon and come back.

I didn't know how I was doing on the test, my mind knew the answers, but I couldn't express them in words. It was a long emotional day. I thought the test would show I was an idiot, even though I knew I wasn't.

Then I tried to explain to her that my right side was numb. I was like a half person. Because I couldn't feel, I'd burn myself, or shut doors on my leg. She didn't believe me, so she came around her desk, put her full weight on me and asked "Do you feel this?" She couldn't understand that I couldn't feel sensations, however I could feel the heaviness of her weight on me. She tried to tell me I was imagining the numbness.

She then set another appointment with me for after the tests were evaluated. I sensed I did badly on the tests even though I knew the answers.

For the next seven days I worked eight hours a day trying to put my treatment plan for myself on paper. Every time I would get a thought it would vanish. I had to get a word and quickly put it down on paper before I'd lose it. I wrote word after word, until I could put them together, attempting to make an outline. Finally I had a very comprehensive plan, which included facts about strokes, along with a time frame. I then wrote, in three years I'll come back, you can test me again, then retrain me if its possible. I need at least three years of therapy before I can even think about retraining. Their money would be better spent on therapy for me, rather than on retraining me for a job I couldn't possibly do at this point in time.

My daughter typed my therapy plan. I took this plan to my next appointment with the psychologist. She wrote a letter to Vocational Rehabilitative Services requesting money for therapy for me. About a month later I received a response from them stating that they had no money for therapy.

CASE CLOSED!

Chapter 7

THE TRIP

During the first week of February, Larry Brown, a colleague of mine, called me from Perry, Florida. Larry worked for Procter and Gamble, he was in charge of the Employee Assistance Program. This was funny to me because two years ago they had wanted me to work for them as the head of this office. I had decided that I didn't want the job, so I didn't bother with the application process.

Larry had called me to come up and sit in his office while he attended a workshop. I told him I didn't know if I could do casework and I definitely couldn't write notes for his clients files. He said all that was required of me was to listen to one former client in process. The rest of the time all I would be responsible for was being there to refer any clients in crisis.

I was skeptical. In spite of feeling very insecure, I desperately needed the money so I decided to go.

Larry took me out to lunch, then over to his apartment where I would be staying. After seeing my accommodations we went to the plant. Some of my ex-clients worked there. I met the nurse and Larry showed me that he had cleared his calendar for me, except for the one former client appointment. I was comfortable with this, although I was worried a crisis might come up. Larry was on his way to his workshop and I was on my own. I visited for awhile with Larry's assistant Al. He took me on a tour of the plant which was in a separate building. I finished out the day and went to Larry's apartment. It was a dark, dreary day; cold and rainy and not at all like the climate in Sarasota. I read a little and went to bed.

The next morning I went to work at eight. It was an uneventful day. I was so bored, I felt as though I had been there three days instead of just one. I did my exercises. One of my clients took me to lunch.

When I went back to the apartment that evening, I found I was lonely. I called Ginger to talk. She and her friend had just got home from having a psychic reading. She told me about her reading. It seemed interesting, until she got to the part about me, he told her that "He is a dead man, Get rid of him!" I asked how he could know. She said he looked at a picture of me. I asked which one, a picture that was taken at Christmas, which I was just coming out of my depression. I told her that at that time I was dead, so I just let the psychic's comment go; or so I thought. I watched some television and went to bed. The feeling of aloneness washed over me and I was feeling cold.

I woke up at four the next morning. I was freaking out. I felt the way I had felt in Fort Myers right before the stroke. I was wondering if they had a hospital here in the small town of Perry. I was so worried that I started to pace.

I was anxious about being there alone, so I lay in the bed with the phone cradled in my arms. I picked up the receiver to call 911 at least five times, hanging it up before I actually dialed the number. One side of me said I was going to have another stroke, while the other side was telling me to calm down; it was just another electrical short circuit in my head. The two sides fought back and forth till I thought my body would rip in two. "Why did I come up here? I don't need or want this," I cried.

By the time I was to report to work I was able to put myself in check. The client came for her appointment. She was there to get help with her anxiety attacks so she could stay off Xanax. Here I was with one Xanax left, to help me with my anxiety attacks. I hoped she wouldn't have an anxiety attack. I need not have worried, she talked about her anxiety while I talked about mine. It was a good session, we both felt good when it was over.

The following day one of the employees from the plant called. He needed to talk to someone. When he arrived at the office I explained to him the situation with my speech. I understood what he needed so I was able to help him with a referral. It was a pretty good day, but I was still feeling alone. I was anxious to go home. I told Al I needed to leave at eleven the next morning. I wanted to make sure he'd be around. The following morning I went to work. I left at eleven so that I would be back in Sarasota before dark. I didn't take the last Xanax, I was feeling okay for the first hour, then my eye started giving me trouble. I had to pull over and relax for fifteen minutes. I closed my eyes, then I drove another half hour. Once again I had to pull over. I was afraid I was going to have to call Ginger to come and get me. I took my last Xanax, and continued on my way. I finally made it home around six. I was so relieved to be home. I talked to Ginger for awhile but I was so tired I went to bed.

When I'm tired and excited, my speech is bad. When I just talk normal, it isn't automatic. When I talk, I have to be conscious of my words, like, If —— I —— speak —— like —— this —— I —— can —— get —— the —— message —— out. The —— problem —— is —— most —— people —— don't —— like —— it —— in —— a —— social —— setting. If I talk normal it's worse because its like this, "They Wkl way an or run an way." (They will walk or run away). I felt that I had to learn more ways of expression.

In May 1993, I was feeling frustrated because I couldn't understand what strokes were about. It seemed that no one knew anything. I then saw an ad at Doctor's Hospital: "Stroke, is it your time bomb?" I went and I received a lot of information. I also noticed that my anxiety level was high as soon as I came into the hospital. As I was listening to the doctors, I could tell that they didn't know much about strokes. I was going to ask, but someone beat me to it. He asked the question, "It appears that the medical establishment doesn't know much about strokes." The doctor agreed. Example, when someone has a heart attack and he can get to the hospital, a team of specialists can save him. With a stroke, they cannot fix it, so your life is in the hands of God. In this country, there are two experimental drugs that will stop some of the damage after the stroke, but they aren't approved at this time.

Chapter 8

EXPRESSION

I was feeling a strong urge to express myself. I felt an inner hesitation or conflict about becoming more creative. There was some kind of internal tension—DAMN, I'm tired of trying to express in words. It seemed as if my brain was responding to the injury, locking it into a self-protective mode of restricted function.

Everyday, I would take an hour to read out loud. I felt the strain on my brain, as if I were pumping iron in the gym. After this I would need to sleep. I had progressed from two sentences in an hour to a page, within a month. But I still didn't know what I had read. When I would speak, some of the words would come out backwards. At times, I had no control of my mouth. At times I felt embarrassed, yet at other times I would feel like a little child, a retarded little child. I thought I was going to be speechless for the rest of my life. I realized at this point, that I had a problem with my short-term memory. This is the memory process used in thought, so when I thought of what I wanted to say, it would be erased. I couldn't type, sing, write or spell anymore. The only means of expression I had was to cry.

The vocational school had a beginning art class. I signed up. In the first class, there were twenty aspiring artists. We started with stick people. I couldn't even draw stick people, I felt totally out of place. At this time I was still having trouble with my vision. I had no control over the focus of my right eye, and boy did that give me perception problems.

However I could see that I could express my feelings on a lower level using simple drawings.

They graduated me from stick people in five minutes. I was just getting into it. I thought I needed more practice. I supposed that the more experienced artists were bored with stick people, so we moved on.

Then we had to make a decision. Five minutes ago I was in kindergarten, then we must have skipped a few grades, because we moved into decision making. We had to decide on something to draw. I didn't know what to draw, the pressure was on. What should I draw? The clock went ticktock, ticktock. I could see that everyone was drawing. Then I had a bright idea. I took one of my shoes off. I put it on the table and proceeded to draw it. I was proud of my drawing. I knew I needed instruction in perception. I was able to learn about perception but I was not able to retain the information. We used different mediums, charcoal, oil paint and water color. I worked on my design at home and completed an oil painting. Looking back at the oil painting I could see where I was then: In the black with anger and only a little light. That painting class was very good therapy for me.

Then I signed up for a class on creating gourds, but I couldn't afford to purchase these gourds, so I thought I would grow my own.

I created my own little gourd patch. I had fun with it. Everyday I was out in my gourd patch fighting the bugs. I talked to them, I reasoned with them, but it didn't work. I didn't want to kill them, so we made a deal, but the bugs broke the deal. I had to save my gourds. I was a general with no troops. Everyday we did battle. I even resorted to chemical warfare. I used numerous chemicals, but their troops kept coming. We battled for three to four months, the bugs suffered huge casualties. When the smoke cleared, I found seven gourds alive. I took my wounded into the house and nurtured them. Then I created each one into an angel. I wanted to continue creating, so I prayed to the head angel. I didn't know if she was going to contact me so I let her go.

Chapter 9

THE PSYCHIC SURGEON

In the Spring of 1993, a friend called me to tell me that The Reverend Alex Orbito was in town. Alex Orbito is a "Psychic Surgeon;" I prefer the term "Spiritual Surgeon." He is from the Philippines but is world famous, having devoted his life to serving humanity. But He does not seek fame. He is renowned as having the gift to heal; however, he quietly has explained himself, saying, "I do not heal. God heals. He uses me only as an instrument for his healing power and forceful energy. I balance the chakra system so that a person can heal himself."

Alex charges no fee for his work, but does accept an offering only if one wishes to pay something. Much has been written by many well-known people about the incredible healing work he has done. I was very skeptical of his unorthodox "surgery" technique. Twenty-five years of counselling had brought me into contact with various "quacks. I am convinced now that his procedure is not quackery, but when I originally encountered Alex Orbito in 1987, had I known what he was about to do to heal my suffering daughter, I may not have chosen the experience because of fear. Not only is it unbelievable, it is impossible to fully describe.

When I was operating The Inner Path, I was having difficulty with creative expression and stress. It seemed to manifest itself with blockage in my neck area. Katie, my daughter, was having some serious medical problems. She was becoming desperate for help and nothing had worked for her. With some trepidation we decided to investigate Alex's recovery procedure.

We went to his healing location and filled out questionnaires. Katie described a cyst about the size of a large olive in her breast which had been noted in her Navy medical records. She also had severe pain in her lower back from a car accident injury and had spent thousands of dollars trying to fix it. I simply wanted him to scan my body to seek and remove any blockage he found.

We went into the room, Alex bowed his head and motioned to Katie to lay on the table. Alex's wife and his assistant sat beside him. Alex went into a deep, silent prayer for awhile. Then he made a mark with his finger nail by the cyst, then he rubbed the skin and took his first two fingers on his right hand and proceeded to push the fingers into the skin. I saw some blood trickle down her body. His fingers were inside of her body past his knuckles, then he put his thumb into her body, and grabbed the lump, pulling it out and threw it in a bowl, it even looked like an olive. When he pulled it out, I could see inside. Then the hole closed, leaving no marks. His assistant and wife washed away the blood with an alcohol gauze. Then he turned her over and went into her lower back and pulled what I considered scar tissue and throwing it into the bowl. Her problems were solved and she hasn't had any problem since.

It was my turn, so I laid on my back. I could feel and see his hand inside my body. It felt like his hand was warm and healing. He pulled out what appeared to be scar tissue from three different areas. Then he went into my throat, he immediately removed his fingers. I sensed that something that I wasn't meant to understand caused him to stop. The session abruptly ended.

I thought about this experience a lot after my stroke and was still unable to comprehend or explain the healing; but I needed some of it. So once again I took a risk, and Ginger drove me down to see Alex.

He was only in town for the weekend, and when we got there, a lot of people were waiting to see him. I hoped he would fix me this time. When it was finally my turn, I went and laid down on the table. I had Ginger write out my slip explaining my dilemma. My experience was exactly the same as it had been six years ago. He put his fingers in my throat and hesitated, as if something warned him to leave it alone. I felt forsaken. I thought maybe there was a reason, maybe I would understand at a later time. However it didn't change the pain I was feeling at this time. I knew now that I would have to do the work, having hope and faith to continue on my journey.

I moved on with my journey. The next step was a neuromuscular therapist! A body worker! WOW! In the early part of my journey I went to a massage therapist. It helped, but, as with everything else, I couldn't afford to continue. Now I had a little income, so I thought if massage had been helpful, I could surely be helped by a neuromuscular body worker. At this point my body was giving me a lot of trouble. My sinuses were plugged twenty-four hours a day. I couldn't breath. I became aware that I was becoming addicted to Afrin. I had started using it before I went to bed, now I was using it three times a day. I felt I needed it, as my usage increased, so did my anxiety attacks. It took all the strength I could muster just to stay on top of the attacks.

I started going to the neuromuscular therapist once a week. It seemed to work, however the relaxed feelings I felt only lasted two days.

As I continued on with this therapy, the deep massages started to trigger some repressed emotional memories. One night after a session, I was so tired I laid down on the floor with my feet up. Soon I was asleep. I had a nightmare, I was under the water struggling, all the while feeling tremendous fear. I couldn't breathe. I felt as though I couldn't hold my breath any longer. I woke up and looked at Ginger. It felt as if my lungs were filled with water. My first thought was, "My father died because there was water in his lungs." I couldn't get my breath. Ginger talked to me. I wanted her to take me to the emergency room. She somehow helped me to get on top of my anxiety. Then I sniffed from my Afrin bottle.

I continued with the neuromuscular therapy for as long as I could, but soon I could not afford it, so I was forced to quit.

Chapter 10

BIOFEEDBACK

It had been one year since my stroke. At this time in my journey, I was aware of getting through the shock and denial. I could see it was a normal process, as a survival mechanism, crucial to my ego's survival. Now I was much more aware of how much damage had occurred. It frightened me. My whole being felt raw, as if all my nerve endings were exposed to the air.

Physically, I looked good. I was walking better than I had before the stroke, thanks to all my exercising, vitamins, my low fat diet, and the fruits and vegetables I ate. My emotional body was a wreck. When I finally came through the shock and denial, the truth finally hit me. This created more emotions, now all I could do was cry. I was at Anabasis that day and had support from the staff. I felt hurt, while at the same time feeling a tremendous sense of loss. I didn't know what to do, I felt so helpless. Mentally I felt no improvement, I was trapped in my mind. Before the stroke I had felt a strong sense of spirit. Now, spiritually, I didn't know. My speech had improved, but I was still having bouts with my anxiety. I had problems with writing and math. It was difficult to focus my right eye. I lacked coordination and balance. My short term memory was bad along with poor concentration. I had tinnitus in my right ear. My right side was still numb. I had become addicted to Afrin. I suffered mild depression, while in the process of grieving all my losses.

This is when I offered myself as a guinea pig at the Biofeedback research lab at Anabasis. I received a grant from Margaret S. Buzzell to support the study of Innovations in the Restoration and Development of the "Sense of Self." I was so miserable with my condition and life, that I wanted to do brain research. I wanted to help myself and in turn hopefully this would help others, to have a better life. This study was not designed as a controlled experimental study. Rather, it was an attempt to facilitate a return to pre-cva functioning, following a non-traditional approach.

The cast in this experiment were James A. Young/the guinea pig, Dr. George Rozelle/scientist, researcher for behavioral medicine at Anabasis, Dr. Tom Budzinski/visiting scholar, scientist at the Center for Behavioral Medicine, University of West Florida, Pensacola, Florida. Timothy W. Hallinan, Ph.D./providing neuromuscular testing. Phyllis Joseph, M.S. C.C.C. and Nelda Foster/speech language pathologists, provided speech evaluations.

I thought about my experiences with Biofeedback, when the lab was started. I couldn't imagine how this would work. When I got to Anabasis and went in, I saw all their new equipment. I didn't understand how it worked, but I was impressed. I had sessions five times a week.

In the beginning we did an initial video tape. They asked me questions, talking and writing. Then they did a two hour brain map. This was interesting. It was in color. I was able to see my brain waves on the computer screen. I didn't understand the dynamics, but the area in my brain that had been damaged was appropriately the color black. After the neuropsychological testing was complete, we were ready to see if I could change my brain waves.

The approach chosen was twofold, combining active and passive feedback techniques. It was called Electroencephalographic Entertainment Feed-Back, (EEF). What a word for someone suffering with aphasia to deal with. I couldn't even say aphasia. I hoped they would give me a test. The authors of this technique hypothesized that it might help to enhance recovery of brain function. "Three stroke victims, 5–7 years after their strokes, began to move again and to recover sensation after sensation." The machine was a little black box, with numerous red lights. It had headphones for programmed rhythmic sounds and stimulation goggles for light. The principle behind this was based on the observed impact on the brain of pulsating lights and rhythmic sounds. Visual stimulus, such as bright light, flickering at a specific rate and an audio tone of the same frequency as the lights stimulus, will cause the brain wave to synchronize with the light stimulus and tone, also appearing to have an entraining effect on the EEG. That was coupled with the computer which printed out the results.

The EEF approach is based on the theory, that in response to an injury, the brain becomes limited in its capability of producing EEF patterns which it cannot change its state to accommodate, changing task demands as easily as before the injury. It appeared that due to the injury, my brain resisted change to protect itself. Hopefully by presenting audio-visual stimuli at varying frequencies, my brain can be retrained or pulled temporarily away from its pathologically limited range of a state allowing a normal reorganization of function to occur. We began; all I had to do was close my eyes and relax. We did four to five sessions per week, for the first twenty-one sessions. During the first session, the light bothered my right eye, the sound bothered my ears. It was as though my brain was telling me to back off. I sensed tremendous resistance. Throughout the first year of this therapy, I felt my brain resisting. As I had learned to speak with my body, I also learned to communicate with my brain.

I continued my old treatment plan of walking three miles each day. I also continued reading out loud everyday. I was lax in my writing because it was so frustrating for me. I couldn't spell. When I had thoughts they vanished. Some of the words were backwards, others were not words at all.

Numerous people were encouraging me to write a book of all my experiences, during this process. They had watched my turnaround and listened to some of my different experiences. They told me that I had helped them. I appreciated their encouragement about writing a book. I thought it would be a wonderful thing to write a book that could help others. But how could I write a book with aphasia, especially with the major amount of brain damage I suffered from the stroke. Damaged brain cells never heal. The brain tissue heals, but only limited improvement, due to reorganization if possible. In my case everyone gave up on me except Teach. She hung on for two more months until her employer pulled her off my case. At this time I couldn't grasp the concept of my writing a book.

I was continuing my daily sessions with light and sound therapy. These sessions were gradually lengthened. I was able to get myself completely relaxed, to the point where I could stay on the line between relaxation and sleep. Some of these times I would slip into sleep. You would think that being relaxed, with nothing to do, I wouldn't feel so exhausted at the end of each session. I would be so tired I would have to go home and sleep.

The light and sound stimulation seemed to be pulling my brain away from its pathology, creating resistance within itself. After twenty-one sessions, there was some improvement, but I had reached a plateau, wherein the EEF stimulation no longer seemed to have any effect on my mental state or functioning. I was becoming bored. My doctor decided to change to a more active neurofeedback procedure.

The goal of the neurofeedback was to decrease the slower frequencies (below 8Hz) and to increase high frequency power. They wired me with electrodes, starting over the central motor control area and later training over the cortical speech areas. I sat in front of what I described as a television monitor. In the center of the screen, was a small oval. On each side of the oval were what looked like thermometers. When I would decrease the slower frequencies on the left thermometer, while at the same time increasing the higher frequency on the right thermometer, the oval would light up green, and produce a pleasant tone. At the same time the counter would count. I had to use my brain to make it work. As I watched my brain waves going up and down in the thermometer, I had little control.

The first of these six sessions were conducted daily. The sessions lasted about an hour. In the beginning, the counter would add up around 40–50. The goal was set to get 500, each session. After a session, I was exhausted. At this time treatment was interrupted for five weeks. Ginger and I decided to go camping.

Before we left for our trip, I had to get my eyes and ears checked. I felt that the trouble I was having with my eyes was causing part of my anxiety. I was referred to an eye doctor. They did some testing and I was told to come back the next day. On the way out I was presented with a bill for $130. I told them I would prefer to wait and pay the total bill tomorrow when I returned. They demanded the payment be made today. The following day the doctor talked to me, stating that there was some damage in my right eye. There was nothing he could do about it. This made me angry, he could have told me this yesterday. He gave me my eyeglass prescription. On the way out I was presented with another bill for $140. I went to get my eyeglasses. This cost me another $250. My money was going out faster than it was coming in. I tried my glasses on, finding only minimal improvement, I became disgusted. My right eye continued giving me problems. Next I went to the ear doctor. He did some testing and told me my ears were okay.

Damn. I thought I would have some relief from my anxiety and feelings of dizziness, especially after spending $800.

Chapter 11

THE CAMPING TRIP

    We were finally able to leave for our five week camping trip. Hopefully we could escape the unbearable heat Sarasota seemed to be engulfed in. Since I had my stroke, I found the heat and sunlight bothered me. Bright light affects my eyes so much, that it was about to drive me crazy. We were going to drive to North Carolina, after which Ginger would be flying to New York for a Yoga workshop. I was going to drop her off at the airport in Atlanta, then I would be driving back to Sarasota by myself.

    We were excited to be going on a trip, because we love to travel together and it's always very peaceful; we also always agree on everything. We were driving a small camper I had.

    We started out heading north. Our first stop would be at Ginger's son's house in Atlanta. The first part of the drive was uneventful. When we drove into Georgia, I felt there was something wrong with the camper. I sensed that I shouldn't drive over 55 miles per hour. When it was Ginger's turn to drive, I felt her speeding up and told her to slow down. I couldn't shake the feeling that something was wrong. We pulled over, I checked the camper over, everything seemed okay, but that foreboding feeling was still there. We finally made it to Atlanta. We had many favorite spots that we enjoyed visiting every time we were in Atlanta. We used Phillip's car both Saturday and Sunday, so I was surprised to find the air conditioner in the camper wasn't working when I went to the store Monday morning. We left downtown Atlanta looking for a shop that could repair it. But because of the extreme heat all of the shops were too busy and didn't have time to fix it. We drove over to Gainesville to the Toyota dealership. With sign language and fragmented speech I pointed out the problems. They said they wouldn't be able to fix it, because it wasn't a Toyota air conditioner, then they referred us to a private shop. They were very nice and more than accommodating to us. They drove us over to the other shop. The man there said that he would be able to fix it. He recommended putting in a transmission cooling system, to keep it cool while were driving through the mountains. We returned to the dealership, then they drove us to a motel, where we watched television and slept. The following morning the Toyota dealer let us borrow a car, while the camper was being fixed. They did so many nice things for us and never charged us a dime. Southern hospitality, it was wonderful.

We drove to Dahlenega in the car they loaned us. Then we drove over to Ellijay; both towns were nice. We wished we could have stayed longer. We had thought it would have been cooler in the mountains, but it wasn't, everyone was saying that this was the hottest summer they had ever had. We drove back to the dealership, only to find out that the camper wouldn't be ready until Wednesday noon. We went back to the motel to spend the night. The next day we picked up the camper at the dealership. We thanked them for everything they had done for us. The owner explained that it was his philosophy to help people, not to rip them off. He tells his employees to bend over backwards to help people. I have never been treated so nicely by strangers in all of my life, and especially not from automobile dealers.

We were going to camp until Friday and then head over to Athens for a wedding we would be attending on Saturday.

We were driving into the mountains looking for a campground. I still had the feeling there was something wrong with the camper. I stopped, got out and looked at the tires, checked everything I could, but nothing appeared wrong. I got back in the camper and continued driving until I found a campground. I backed the camper into our spot, got out and walked around the front of the camper. That's when I noticed one of the front tires was split open about three inches. After that, it seemed to be one thing after another. I decided to put the spare on, so I jacked up the camper, and got the tire off. When I went to put the spare on, I discovered that the rim wouldn't fit. I put the split tire back on, not knowing if I would be able to make it back to town. Although it was hard for me, I put it out of my mind and didn't worry. By doing this, I was able to enjoy my evening. The next morning, after we broke camp, we drove down the road at five miles per hour, hoping to make fifteen miles to the next town. We pulled into a station, but because we didn't have an appointment, they only had time to put a different rim in the spare so that we would be able to use the camper.

The next morning we went back and I bought two heavy duty tires for the front. Now I thought everything was working good.

We went higher into the mountains, where it was cooler. We camped there that night, driving to Athens the next day. After we attended the wedding and reception, we drove on toward North Carolina. That night we camped at a gorgeous lake on the border of Georgia and North Carolina.

The following day we were exploring some back roads, when we saw a sign that said Gourd Museum. I got excited, maybe my prayer to the gourd's angel was answered. We went to the museum. They had a lot of unique creations out of gourds. I questioned the woman, wondering where she had gotten all her gourds. She told me she had gotten them from the "Gourd Lady." Then she gave me the gourd lady's name and address, along with her phone number. She lived in Wren, Georgia, which was quite a ways from where we were. I thought "I'll go there after I drop Ginger off in Atlanta."

We drove up to North Carolina, exploring the back roads as we drove. We explored for a month and were going to go to Atlanta. We went to Highlands, spending that night at a motel. The next morning I went out to get some batteries out of the camper. While trying to reach over everything for the batteries, I slipped and fell, hurting my lower back. I went to a chiropractor for three treatments, but they didn't seem to help. I could barely sit down, let alone drive. Ginger drove us back to Atlanta. Once we were there, Ginger called the airline, explaining the situation. They allowed her to change her ticket so she could drive me back to Sarasota and take a flight from there.

Ginger drove me back to Sarasota. I got some more chiropractic treatments and Ginger flew off to New York.

When Ginger returned from New York with her Yoga Teachers certificate, she asked me to be her student, so she could practice teaching techniques on me. This type of yoga is called Hatha yoga, which uses exercises involving breathing, stretching and balancing. The first class I found to be difficult. However, I could see that it would benefit my recovery. As I continued every week I was able to do more of the different exercises. It helped me with my balance and also healed my back. I was still having trouble with my immune system and was experiencing a lot of congestion. Everyday it seemed as if I was affected by everything. I felt miserable. I told the doctor, but he couldn't help me. All I could do was go through it and have faith. My whole being was affected.

I was now going to biofeedback three times a week. We taped another video in order to evaluate my speech and writing. We repeated the same tests that had been performed for the first video. We wanted to compare the two videos, seeing if I had made any improvement. Although I had made significant improvement in my speech, there appeared to be no improvement in my writing. I was still having problems with losing my thoughts, this in turn caused me to have problems with spelling.

I experimented with different techniques, so I would be able to control my brain waves. I tried my breathwork, so that I could get myself to a relaxed trance like state. By doing this I found that I could control my brain waves better. I also tried to visualize my brain waves going up and down. This appeared to help slightly. Out of all the techniques I employed, the one that worked the best was my being able to put myself in a trance. I was proud of myself, but by staying in a trance, I wouldn't be able to function in any other capacity. I guess I could be a guru and have someone take care of my body while I stayed in a trance. I discussed this with George and he told me to redefine relaxed to mean being in a restful state, but to remain alert and conscious. I found I had to work on being relaxed, while at the same time doing a task. I continued to practice using visional techniques to change my brain waves.

The bookkeeper from Anabasis called. Her husband had suffered a stroke during the night and was in the hospital. I didn't know him, but I thought I would go to the hospital to let him know he wasn't alone. My speech was still bad, but I would do the best I could, hoping that he could understand me.

Ginger drove me to the hospital that evening. We parked in the parking ramp, and started walking towards the door to the hospital. I was fine until we entered the hospital, then my body started reacting. I was feeling apprehension, and my eye was refusing to focus. I knew that I really didn't want to be there. We continued to the room and I was introduced to her husband Jose. I heard his name, but couldn't say it. Soon I forgot his name, and I was too embarrassed to ask her to repeat it. I knew I would soon forget it again anyway. I thought, "What am I doing here?"

He was paralyzed on his right side and he couldn't speak. This appeared to frustrate him. I understood the feeling only too well. I was extremely uncomfortable, while at the same time feeling tremendous compassion for him. I talked to him about my stroke, along with all the anger and frustration that I had felt. It was difficult for me to convey all of this because I was having problems with my speech. My body seemed to be reacting in sympathy to what he was going through. After awhile he was getting tired, so we left. I was never so relieved as I was at that moment and I was so glad to be out of there. I felt I never should have gone in the first place. I felt like a failure. Who was I trying to kid? I was having trouble helping myself. How could I possibly think that I would be able to help anybody else?

A few days later, I found out that he had gotten his speech back when he woke up that morning. The whole problem with his speech had disappeared. This made me feel as though I was doing something wrong in my treatment program. He had gotten his speech back in three days. Why did I seem to be having such a problem. I decided that it was my fault that I hadn't completely recovered my speech yet. So I beat myself up for the next few days.

A few weeks later, I went over to his house and he thanked me for seeing him in the hospital. He stated that it helped him. I asked how his speech came back so fast. He replied "I prayed to God." I thought to myself, "So did I." I was envious. The question, "What was I doing wrong?" kept coming up in my mind as if it was branded in my brain.

I received a message from a speech therapist from Home Health Services, who had worked with me one day while Teach was away. She wanted me to meet her at one of her client's homes. He had aphasia and didn't want to cooperate with her. His progress had stopped at this point. She was hoping that I would somehow be able to help.

The following afternoon Ginger drove me to the client's home. I felt I needed her there to support me, just in case I might fall apart.

The speech therapist introduced us. He was able to walk, but suffered severe aphasia. I talked to him, relating my experiences to his. Looking in his eyes produced a mirrored image of myself. I saw myself so clearly in his eyes that it frightened me. When he spoke it came out gibberish. I knew the frustration he was feeling, for I felt it too. It hurt me to see someone in that kind of pain, not knowing if what I've related to them will be of any help. While sitting there looking into his eyes I felt a deep compassion for him, at the same time feeling powerless. I was having trouble trying to understand my own aphasia, yet I was going out trying to help others. By doing this I was creating more problems within myself.

After we returned home, I spotted a book lying on the coffee table. It was titled "Strokes: What Families Should Know." I picked it up and opened it to a page that read, "No two strokes are ever alike. You'll never know what to expect." This made me feel a little better. I decided to stop trying to help others until I could get myself better.

Chapter 12

THE BREAKUP

For some time, I had been sensing that my relationship with Ginger was on and off. It seemed that it was wonderful a lot of the times, even though I was having anxiety attacks, speech and eye problems and I was a lot slower, we still were active doing things that we enjoyed; little trips, theater, movies, dining out, parties, active sexual life, and feeling of closeness. I was independent and so was she. Then at times, I seemed to feel an undertow of energy that would turn the relationship off. I tried to figure it out. My income went from $35,000 to $10,000, and while that affected the relationship, that wasn't it. I couldn't figure it out. For a number of months, numerous friends were splitting or divorcing, actually there were seven of them. At that time, I remember thinking it was like a contagious disease and I was hoping we wouldn't catch it. Maybe we got it.

The relationship got to the point that it was very uncomfortable living in Ginger's house. We talked about this, deciding that I would move to the other side of the house. The house is set up with two bedrooms and a bath on one side, with the master bedroom and bath on the other. The living room, dining room, and kitchen were in the center, with a lanai running the length of the living room and dining room. By me moving to the other side our relationship changed. Now I was just a renter with kitchen privileges. Then for awhile, the relationship was going on and off. I found living this way made me even more uncomfortable. I didn't know how to behave. I felt as though I were walking on egg shells. It seemed that Ginger was having the same feelings. We talked about many different aspects of our situation. These talks included money. Was I going to get any better? Why couldn't it be the way it used to be? We talked and cried together, giving me feelings of closeness that made me love her even more and it seemed to make her fearful. Everything was confusing to me. My mind tried to sort everything out. My mind went back to the way our relationship had been from the beginning. It was wonderful. We were happy, active, loving, adventurous and travelers. Before my stroke we found it easy to express our feelings, negative or positive.

I was crushed. This was another loss for me. I felt like an orange being squeezed until no juice remained in the skin. It was as though with each drop of juice, the empty feelings of my losses kept mounting, until I was just a shell of a man. I was having a hard time letting go. Somehow this had to be a purification process, by letting go of everything in my life.

Ginger was becoming more and more busy. It was as though she didn't want to come home. This led me to feel guilty. I felt she wasn't coming home because I was there. Because it was her house, I felt like an intruder.

Finally we sat down and talked; we decided that it would be best if I would move out and rent a room somewhere else. She said I could take my time. I didn't like the uncomfortable guilty feelings I was experiencing. They made me feel like running, somewhere—anywhere—it didn't matter. I immediately started looking at rooms. The better rooms were renting for $400 to $500 per month and I knew I couldn't afford this along with my food and medical bills. As the search continued, feelings of desolation were beginning to overcome me. I finally found some cheaper rooms, but they were in the ghetto. I had a fear that if I rented one of these, I would end up being stuck there for the rest of my life. I felt depression would soon overcome me if I was forced to live there.

I continued searching, each day brought only discouragement. This discouragement, along with my pain and grief, was tying my stomach into knots, twisting, churning, tightening, like tree roots gnarling around. My emotional pain was causing this physical pain, tearing me up. I had to run, but where? I couldn't afford much. I was like an animal caught in a trap, trying to chew my leg off so I could escape.

I have always felt a lot of compassion for the homeless. Now it looked as though I would become one, wandering around trying to find a spot for myself. Because I had a small camper, I felt my only alternative was to live in it. I called my daughter Laurie, I wanted her to go look at campsites with me. I hadn't realized that because we were going into the winter tourist season, that the campgrounds charge a higher price. We looked at several sites. It would have cost me double what a room would cost. Beside the $465 a month for the campsite, I would have to pay for my electricity, costing $60 a week, plus a $15 dumping fee each time I had to dispose of my waste. I couldn't believe it, I would have to pay through the nose, just to rough it. Talk about survival! I knew this was out of the question. I drove Laurie home and was feeling only despair as I returned to Ginger's house. Once again I was studying the classifieds looking for a room to rent. Finally I felt so desperate, that I started looking for a room in another town, where it was less expensive. I found a room for $350 a month. It was a nice room and I liked the people. I went back to Ginger's house to pack and move. Throughout the move, all we could do was cry. I asked Ginger about rights with the children, Lucy and Tiger; she smiled.

Once I moved into my new room, I found it difficult living there. I had to drive to Sarasota everyday for my biofeedback, doctor appointments and other activities. I'd go to Sarasota everyday, returning to my room at night, where I lay licking my wound, trying to heal it. I had freed myself from one trap only to become ensnared in a web. The grass was not greener on the other side of the fence. Because it was someone else's home, I felt like a guest. My feelings of despair and grief hadn't diminished. I had traded one set of living circumstances for another, thinking I could run from my problems. I knew I needed my independence. But how? I still had no money. I felt stuck and I knew running would do me no good.

I felt I needed a place for myself. How could I do this? This one thought occupied my mind constantly. I was still trying to find a way, when Ginger called. She was thinking about doing something with me for my birthday. She wanted to know if I wanted to take a trip to Wren, Georgia to see the Gourd Lady, then maybe drive over to Charleston for a few days. I agreed that it would be a nice thing to do. She also wanted to know if I would baby-sit Lucy and Tiger for a week. I jumped at the chance to be back in Sarasota, even if it was only for a week.

Once at Ginger's house, I started looking in the classifieds again. I got excited when I read an ad for a free trailer. I immediately called Laurie. She called the number for me to find out what the deal was. When she finally called back, she told me that the trailer was in bad shape. It was free to someone, if they would fix it up and sign a lease agreeing to rent the lot in their adult park for three years. Then the trailer would be mine.

The next morning we went to look at the trailer. Even though the manager had warned us, we were a little disappointed in how bad it really was. The floor was rotted through in three places. The ceiling was full of water, where the roof had leaked, and everything inside was damaged. It was so bad that about one hundred people had looked at it and turned the offer down. But it was free and I thought with a little work, I could make it livable. I didn't realize what I was getting myself into. If I had, I would have been afraid to take the risk.

Two days later we went back and I signed the lease agreement. The manager gave me two months free lot rent. We also discussed my handy man skills and she told me that if I laid carpet for them when they needed it done that I could get some more lot rent free. This sounded good to me. Laurie and I went over to the trailer to figure out where we would start. I ripped away some rotted wood and saw that the trailer was infested with termites. Laurie called a friend of hers and made arrangements to have it tented while I was on my birthday trip with Ginger. The manager gave me an extra months free lot rent, because I needed to have it tented. The next day we were at the trailer, clearing everything out, so we could get started when I returned from my trip. They came to tent it and I returned to Ginger's house, getting my things packed so Ginger and I could leave in the morning.

Chapter 13

THE GOURD LADY

We left at 8 A.M. and we arrived at 5 P.M. the same day. The Gourd Lady's farm was in a small farming community, located outside of Wren, Georgia. As we drove up a long gravel driveway, it appeared that the farm was about 150 acres. The Gourd Lady raised just gourds for people like me to use for creations. In front of the house was a tree with green gourds lying under it. Along the front of all of this, platforms were stretching for acres. These were filled with gourds drying in the sun. Being surrounded by all these gourds, filled me with excitement. The head angel really answered my prayer in a big way. I silently thanked her. I felt I had died and gone to gourd heaven.

We walked up and down the rows of gourds examining all of them. Greed had overtaken me, I wanted all of them. I felt like a child in a candy store, Ginger got hooked and was grabbing gourds for herself. This is what we do when we travel: we have fun. Any thought or feeling I had of our breakup vanished. We were having visions of what we would create with each gourd.

Reality finally hit. How was I going to pay for all of these gourds? I didn't even know how much the Gourd Lady charged. I ran to the house and knocked. She came out, I wanted to deal, but I was having difficulty communicating with her. When I'm tired, my speech regresses back to the early days of my recovery. My words were twisted. She couldn't understand what I was trying to say. This embarrassed me. When this happens, it makes my speech worse. Through persistence, I was finally able to make a deal on the price. The Gourd Lady accepted 50 cents for each gourd.

Ginger was still out in the field picking out gourds and I joined her. We had over one hundred gourds. My entrepreneur self kicked in, I was thinking, I could come up here to pick up gourds, then bring them back to Sarasota and sell them for five to eight dollars a piece, compared to the ten to fifteen dollars that the gourds sold for in Sarasota.

Ginger and I were pleased with ourselves. We had a haul. We felt like children who had gotten an overwhelming amount of presents at Christmas time. Then we found a motel room and went to dinner.

The next morning we were heading southeast on our way to Charleston. We stopped a few times along the way for some sight-seeing. This was a pleasant and peaceful trip.

We had made reservations at a bed and breakfast in downtown Charleston, a block away from the ocean. We checked in that afternoon. We went up to our room, enjoying the Spanish decor. There was a bedroom and a living room with a balcony that overlooked a courtyard. We found it very comforting and peaceful and we relaxed for a bit. Around dinner time we took a walk and found a nice restaurant, filled with 18th century antiques. We had dinner there, enjoying the atmosphere. I was having trouble with my speech so Ginger ordered for me. I had trouble with the fact that I was the man and should be ordering for her. However, this was soon forgotten in this wonderfully relaxing, peaceful atmosphere.

After dinner, we strolled hand in hand down to the boardwalk that ran along the ocean. The sun was setting in the west allowing splashes of color to highlight the sky. Fishermen were fishing, lovers were kissing, children were playing. It was as though we were in a storybook setting not having a care in the world. We stopped to talk to a young couple. It felt like a family get together. The atmosphere seemed to bring people together. We started back to the bed and breakfast. My fondest memories of the city came back to me. I remember wanting to move there when I had visited Katie. As we strolled back to the bed and breakfast, I didn't want the evening to end. I slept peacefully throughout the night.

The following morning, breakfast was brought up to our balcony. As we sat eating our breakfast, the sun was just starting to peak over the horizon. As it rose up into the sky its light shown across the water, making everything sparkle. It was so beautiful that it brought a feeling of peacefulness across the city.

After breakfast, we went to explore downtown. We walked admiring all the beautiful old historical buildings. We went to the open market, there were hundreds of vendors selling their wares. We explored the old train station. We found Charleston filled with history. Most of the day was spent exploring. Too soon it was time to move on.

We were on our way to Buford. We were traveling down the back roads trying to get to Interstate 19. The sun was setting and we soon found ourselves in darkness. The quietness with the darkness on that back road gave us feelings of uneasiness. It was as though an eeriness blanketed the countryside. The further we traveled, it seemed that maybe we were lost. Ginger saw an I-19 sign. I stopped, the sign pointed down a dark narrow road, I could see lights in the distance ahead, so we were debating which road to take. Our imagination started working overtime. We decided that someone had turned the sign around and that they were waiting at the end of the road to ambush us leaving us for dead. It was amazing that our minds think the same thoughts. We decided to go toward The Light. Finally we made it to the highway. We had spooked ourselves so bad, we stopped to spend the night at a motel to give our imaginations time to unwind.

The next morning, we left to continue on our way to Buford. We walked around this charming little town, then sat on a bench to view the marshland while listening to the birds. We were amazed at the amount of wildlife there.

It was time to go home, even though we were tired, I would have liked to continue traveling. We took turns driving back to Sarasota. Another wonderful birthday present.

I spent that night at Ginger's house. The following morning I went to my trailer. The pest control company hadn't taken the tent off of the trailer, so I decided to take the day off.

Chapter 14

A HOME FOR ME

Now was the beginning of a major creation. I was able to go into my trailer. It was a hovel. I just looked at it. Oh! My God! Maybe the Goodwill trailer job would have been easier. I had sold most everything I had so that I would have some money to put into the trailer. We started hauling the junk out of the trailer. We worked all day: Laurie hauled trash, I ripped the ceiling down. As I tore through the roof, buckets of water came down, filling the floor with two inches of it. Now I could see what was needed to fix the roof.

That evening as I sat planning, I started to make a list of things we would need from Home Depot. This was difficult for me, because of my aphasia. The words I wrote down were all jumbled. I wanted 2" X 2" X 8' long studs, but could not get it down on my list, so I wrote down sticks.

The next morning Laurie came to pick me up to go to Home Depot to get our supplies. Laurie looked at my list and because she knew most of what we needed, she understood most of what I had written on my list. There were a few words that she couldn't make out and had no idea of what I had written. This was the beginning of our learning to communicate with little or no words. We drove to Home Depot, hoping I would remember what I had written when we got there.

Once at Home Depot we got a big cart and started to fill it with the things on our list. While going through the store, we saw all sorts of tools that we thought would be nice to have, but I couldn't afford them. At this time we thought in terms of fixing the trailer. We thought that we would make do with the tools we had. These tools consisted of a measuring tape, hammer, drill and two screwdrivers. The only other tool I bought at this time was a hand saw to cut my sticks. We spent most of the day at Home Depot. On the way home we stopped to eat. While we were eating we made plans for the trailer. Then we went back to the trailer, unloading what we had bought. I was disappointed because we hadn't gotten anything done at the trailer and it was almost time for Laurie to leave. Before Laurie left, she made a list of things to bring from home, including a crow bar and extension cord.

The next morning I got up at five and was working by seven. I wanted to get the roof started. This is a 1960 "New Moon." The roof was sunk in, so I used my studs to begin to raise it up. I was able to push the tin up and slide my 2" X 2" stud in the center. I went from the front to the back. My thoughts were to use the sun's heat to stretch the tin and at three or four in the afternoon, when it was the hottest time of the day, I would push another stud on top of the first. It took a couple of weeks to stretch the tin.

Laurie came over and continued hauling the junk out. As the days wore on the pile of junk in the carport grew higher and higher. I started to wonder what I had gotten myself into. Laurie started loading her station wagon with the junk, taking load after load over to the dumpster. Soon the dumpster was full, yet there was still a huge amount of garbage piled up in the carport. We were exhausted, so Laurie went home, leaving me sitting in a pile of junk that I was soon to call my home. All that evening, I planned where I needed to start and what materials I would need to get started. I was dirty and tired. Thankfully I was able to use the shower in the trailer. I cleaned myself up so I could go get something to eat.

After dinner, I sat in the trailer to plan my next move. Then I went to sleep at 9 P.M. in the camper. The next morning I continued to work on the roof and Laurie hauled junk. In the afternoon I worked on the floor and found that I had trouble with measuring. I would measure and I would forget what I had just measured. This started to make me frustrated. Then I tried to write it down. I would measure 2' X 4' and would write a different number down. After a while, I started to make a mark on my ruler and take my ruler and mark the board. Then after a while, there were to many marks on the ruler and it was messing me up. Things that I had done before the stroke eluded me now.

I began in the bedroom and bath, because I wanted to finish them so I could move out of the camper into the back of the trailer. Laurie left to pick up a microwave oven for me from her girlfriend. I went to take my shower and as I was taking my shower, suddenly, I was in motion.

With one hand on the wall, the other grabbing the sink, the tub started to fall through the rotted floor beneath. My adrenaline level shot up and fear swept through me as the tub hit the ground. I was amazed I wasn't hurt. There I stood, the man in the can with no shower curtain. My feet were on the ground, my knees were at the level of the floor and the rest of my body was in the bathroom, so I just continued finishing my shower as if nothing had happened. I was amused and had to chuckle at myself standing there knee high to the bathroom floor. After I finished, I went to the Manager's office. They said I could use their shower as long as I needed to.

My brain wasn't with it while fixing the floor in the bedroom and the kitchen. It hadn't even occurred to me that the floor might be rotted from the bedroom to the kitchen which would include the floor under the tub.

The next day, I ripped the wall down where the tub was, to find that the two by two's were rotted away, there wasn't a wall. Then I discovered the old wiring, I picked up one of the wire's and it crumbled in my hands. It frightened me. At that time, I decided that I would rip everything out down to the metal. When we got finished, I decided to create a house inside of the metal, so when you are outside, it looks like a trailer, when you come in and close the door, you're in a house. That began making people notice. Everyday people from the park came to tell me that I can't do this in a trailer. You can't use sheet rock. You can't put ceramic tile in the bathroom. You can't put ceramic tile on the floor. You can't. You can't. You can't——. That gave me the strength that I was going to need to complete my creation.

Every day, seven days a week, we labored. The roof was stretched and braced solidly. Outside it looked like a covered wagon, inside I had raised the roof ten inches, giving me ten inches of insulation. Laurie put the first coat of "cool white" on the roof, then the rain came, continuing on throughout the night.

In the middle of the night, I woke up soaked. My camper was leaking. I was disgusted and went into the trailer, to find puddles on the floor. The roof was still leaking in spots. Every night it rained, every day we kept finding puddles on the floor. It was getting old after a while. It seemed as if we're going through the famous flood in Genesis, "The water continued forty days and forty nights. God said to

Noah, make yourself an ark."

One Friday, as the rain continued, I met Ginger for a yoga workshop. I was telling her about the problems I was having with my camper and trailer, so she offered to let me stay in her extra room, so I worked in the day and slept at night there. By then I was tired of the rain. I was frustrated, but the rain found places that we couldn't, consequently it was a positive note.

The next Thursday I quit early and went to Ginger's house for her Yoga class. We were talking, I don't remember what about, but it brought up the subject of my depression. I felt a lot of anger coming up from my stomach. I screamed at her. I said I don't believe the depression was the reason that we split and if it was, I couldn't help it. I tried to settle down, but my anger kept coming. I decided to get out of there and go back to the trailer, and sleep in my camper. It was the end of October and I decided that it is over. I didn't call her or see her. She didn't call me either. I was hurting bad, it was like someone blew a huge hole into the center of my stomach and heart that went all the way through coming out through my back. It seemed as if the wind was blowing through the hole, hitting every nerve.

The next month, Laurie and I worked every day trying to finish the bedroom and bathroom. Most of this time I was in a daze. I was having a hard time dealing with the loss of Ginger. I mourned for the old days. I was throwing myself into my work, but the grief and mental anguish I was feeling was constantly present. Now my concentration was even worse. Laurie was frustrated with me, so she worked by herself on different projects in the trailer, only helping me when I asked for help. While I would be working on one thing, I would forget what I was doing, wandering off to do something else. By the middle of November, we had somehow set up a system between us. This system left me working by myself most of the time, giving me the chance to try to get over my loss. I hadn't dealt with the loss of the relationship from the beginning, because I didn't want to feel this pain. I knew now that I would have to deal with it no matter how painful it was or I would never be able to move on with my life. At night, I would cry, by day I worked on my creation, it was a tool to express my feelings.

I ran all of the new wire for the electrical system. I bought a circuit breaker box and hung it in the closet. I wanted to go all electric, so I put twelve circuits in it. When I would start a wire from the box, I would write a note showing where it was going and attach it to the wire. The problem was I couldn't read my notes. I struggled to figure a way to do it as I sat there, I thought about drawing a symbol, like bedroom air conditioner, I used B/Air. I drew the stove and refrigerator, I drew a light bulb over the table, etc. It took me three days just to run the wires in the ceiling. Before my stroke, I would have been finished in a day. I was thinking about the old circuits and wires and related it to my electrical system in my brain. I guess I was putting all new wires in my home and also into my brain.

We were discouraged at the amount of time it was taking us to accomplish each task. Finally we were able to see some progress.

The nights were getting colder and I was having a hard time controlling the heat in the camper. After a short time it would become too hot, so I'd turn the heater off, then it would become cold. My right side ached from the cold and I had trouble working.

We were hoping to have the bedroom finished by Thanksgiving. (Note, it does get cold in Florida, in November, December and January having temperatures in the thirties.) I had to go to my yearly ultrasound checkup. When I was having this checkup, she told me that my body wasn't producing the plaque. I also went to get my yearly physical and I was in good shape.

We continued to finish the bedroom and bathroom. I insulated the walls and ceiling and we were hanging sheet rock. I had trouble using my right hand to cut the sheet rock. My hand would move off the straight edge, so I tried to visualize, with my eyes open, my hand going down the straight edge and it seemed to help.

The park was having an early Thanksgiving dinner so we stopped early so I could go. I enjoyed the dinner and met new people. While at the dinner, everyone talked me into going to Bingo, so I decided to try it. Everyone had fifteen cards in front of them, I had one. The caller would say "I 21". By the time my mind would register I 21, the caller would say "B 3". I was still thinking I 21, consequently I would miss B 3 and then the caller would be on N 23. I just couldn't keep up; so people were helping me, which made me feel embarrassed. After a while some assumed that I was just fooling around and being funny. I said, "Give me a break, I have a lot of brain damage." This made them laugh, so I quit. As I was walking back to my camper, I thought that maybe Bingo would be good therapy, trying to coordinate letters and numbers. Even though I thought about Bingo as a therapy, I never went back. Maybe because I had seen it as an old farts game. I remembered when Ginger and I went to Costa Rica on a white water rafting trip, a twenty-three year old guy, who ran the raft talked to us at lunch. He was very serious and said, "My dream is to retire, move to Florida, get a trailer and play shuffleboard and Bingo." That is not my cup of tea.

Thanksgiving was here and I was still in the camper. I got to thinking about Ginger and the past Thanksgiving on the farm in Fort Myers and how we always had a good time. Soon I went to sleep. I woke up Thanksgiving day even more depressed than I had been the day before. Laurie had invited me to her house for dinner, but I had turned her down. I guess I didn't want to be in a happy festive environment. I was still trying to deal with all of my losses. My emotional state was in turmoil. The sky was overcast, blanketing the city in dreariness. The temperature had dropped, making the wind feel like icy fingers trying to grab hold of me. The weather of the day lowered my spirit even more.

One of my neighbors had invited me to the Salvation Army for their Thanksgiving meal. I decided I would go rather than stay home feeling miserable. When we got there I focused my attention on the many children that were there with their parents. Quite a few had no homes and were living in their cars. I felt like crying. The compassion I felt for these children was overwhelming. What kind of chance would they have for the kind of life that would give them a feeling of security?

As we stood in line waiting to be served, I talked to the homeless, and to those who could not afford food. Everyone of them was grateful. They were thankful for the volunteers and everyone who made this dinner possible. Everyone was in good spirits. I appeared to be the only one full of sadness.

After eating, I talked for a while with the volunteers. I gave them a donation and headed home feeling better than I had all month. By focusing on their high spirits in spite of their problems, I was somehow lifted out of my self pity.

When I got home, I put on my work clothes, hoping to accomplish something on the trailer. I didn't get much done, but I was feeling better so it didn't bother me.

Each day the bedroom was coming to a completion. I tiled the bathroom; with only one mistake, it turned out well. My right arm and hand were cumbersome, so I was dropping the tiles. Some would break, but all in all it was making me feel better. Now the creation was starting to show itself.

I was ready to start sleeping in the trailer. I bought some floor heaters. A woman down the street let me borrow a double wide air mattress to sleep on. That night I found that I was still cold even though the bedroom was warm. I hadn't thought about the air in the mattress staying cold because of the lack of insulation in the floor. I had to put blankets on the bottom and on top of me. I decided that the day before Christmas, I would buy a new bed, which would be here within two weeks.

The day before Christmas, we went shopping. I had picked out my bed a few days before, so all I had to do was pay for it. Then Laurie and I shopped and bought two lamps, two night stands, along with sheets, pillows and a comforter. I felt good, I was able to push my pain aside, allowing me to ignore it—even if it was only for the day. All I could think about was how nice it would be sleeping in my brand new bed. I went to bed that night happy.

I woke up the next morning feeling pretty good. Laurie was going to be gone, so I thought I would go back to the Salvation Army for dinner. Before dinner I was feeling lonely, but it passed when I went to the Salvation Army. I got through Christmas, my pain was easing. I continued working on my house.

By January 1, 1994, my trailer was becoming a house. I still missed Ginger, but I wasn't in so much pain. Laurie and I completed the kitchen and dining room and were working in the living room.

I was faithfully continuing with my biofeedback and I felt that it was helping. The resistance that I felt in the past months was getting less. I asked George to let me see the tape we made last June. The tape was made one year after the stroke. As I watched the tape and saw myself as an old, slumped and haggard man who stumbled over his words, it made me cry. My mind told me that I looked good. As I was crying, I thought, God, no wonder Ginger had to run. I looked like death warmed up; I probably would have run too. After I viewed the tape, I was talking with one of my colleagues, when all of a sudden everything that I had accumulated in my emotional body over the past fifteen months came out. Tears burst forth, gushing from my eyes flooding my face. I just cried and cried. The staff at Anabasis were very supportive throughout my catharsis. The reality hit me, my brain was damaged and I couldn't undo it. I knew I would have to learn to accept and deal with it, while at the same time not giving up and pitying myself. I took a couple of days off and rested.

One day one of my neighbors who came to see me daily brought his wife over to meet me. When she spoke I had a feeling deep within me, a voice said, "She is having a stroke." I asked her how she was feeling. She said that she was having dizziness, double vision, headaches and numbness in her right side. I asked if she had seen a doctor. She replied that she went to an eye doctor but he didn't know what her problem was. I said, I think that you are having a stroke and I gave her husband the number of my neurologist. He called and found that they couldn't get an appointment until January 14. No one seemed too worried, so I continued to work on the trailer. I didn't think anymore about it.

It took her a month before she was admitted to the hospital. When she came home, she couldn't speak, but was able to walk. She came over daily and sat in a chair in a stupor. I talked to her daily giving her support. After awhile, her husband called us frick and frack. A month later she had to go back to the hospital for more surgery. Soon she was back, starting to recover. She went to a speech therapist for a few months and then was on her own.

Chapter 15

SEARCHING FOR A NEW SELF

    One day, Ginger came to the trailer. I hadn't spoken to her for three months. I gave her a tour of my home, then we sat down and talked. I still had deep feelings in my heart for her. Pretty soon we were dating again. She was going to Costa Rica for a week to see our friends who moved there. I took her to the airport in Tampa and it brought up some feelings about our travels. I was envious and sad because I wasn't going to fly with her.

    By February my trailer was coming to a completion, and I began to think in terms of, "What was I going to do with my life?" By now, I had put myself in further debt, and I didn't know how to make a living. My profession that I loved and did well in was out of the question. It required paperwork, and I couldn't write, spell, and put sentences together. My speech had improved tremendously, but not to the point of doing the job. I wanted to get back to creating things with my gourds, hopefully I could sell them. In the meantime, to get instant cash, maybe I could be a handyman! I went to a printer to get some cards printed, "The Handi-Man Can." I proceeded to promote my business. I put cards around the trailer park and on the Key. I was still doing carpet installation in the trailer park to get my lot rent paid for and was starting to get business on the key.

    Ginger called, asking me if she could hire me to convert her garage into a yoga studio. I accepted and part of the deal was to let me be one of the students, one night a week. Since Ginger and I parted, I missed the yoga exercises, so I was trying to find another studio. I had a number of jobs scheduled, but I was able to fit Ginger's studio in my schedule. Everything seemed to fall together leaving me some time to create my gourds.

    In the beginning, it was okay; but physically I was beginning to have problems with my right leg, arm, and my right eye was still giving me trouble. It was one thing to work on my trailer, another to work for someone else. First, Laurie wasn't there to help. Second, I couldn't lay down when I was hurting. Third, my customers noticed me wandering around in a stupor, at times forgetting what I was doing. I would measure five times to cut a board, often dropping my tools on the floor. At times it appeared that I didn't know what I was doing because of my clumsiness. Fourth, I was still plagued with anxiety attacks and once in awhile I would have one so I would go to my truck and breathe. My customers were paying me by the hour, consequently I wasn't getting referrals to build the business. I completed all of the carpet jobs that I contracted for, slowly my business was nil.

I continued creating my gourds, everyone admired them but no one bought any. I was okay with that, because I felt like creating the gourds was helping in my recovery, using my creative brain.

One morning, I woke with a tremendous pain in my left shoulder that ran up my neck. My mind raced, trying to figure out what was happening. I was able to dissipate some of the anxiety with my breathing exercises.

I lay in bed clutching my shoulder, crying in agony. I didn't know what to do. Then it dawned on me to call my friend who is a chiropractor. I went to his home where he massaged and manipulated my shoulder. He was able to loosen the tightness. Although it felt better when he was finished, later in the day, it was hurting again. I went back and he adjusted me again. This went on for two days, with more adjustments and using aspirin for the pain. Still the pain continued. Someone said that I was experiencing arthritis, which I couldn't do anything about. On the third day, after a long restless night, I decided to go to the doctor. I was sitting in bed and I got to thinking about my training in Alchemical/Hypnotherapy. One of the many exercises I learned was to hypnotize myself. My plan was to hypnotize myself, count down ten steps, open a door and step into the pain. I was able to relax myself as I went down the steps, opened the door and stepped into the pain. Then I was an Indian running across an open field. I had an arrow stuck in my left shoulder. My present body was feeling so much pain, I thought that I would pass out. As the Indian fell onto the ground, his mate came running. She pulled the arrow out of my shoulder. The pain was excruciating. After awhile my pain was gone. As the Indian, I looked into my mate's face. It was Ginger. I didn't try to analyze it. All I knew was that the pain was gone.

That morning, I created a gourd that has a face of an eagle and within the center of the face is an Indian. Everyday that I was creating, I felt free and joyful, but deep inside there was something pushing me.

I longed to do what I did best, helping people. One morning, while I was doing my daily walk, a car pulled over to the curb. It was a friend whom I hadn't seen for some time. She is a therapist in the Alcohol/Drug Dependent business. We talked awhile about where she was working. She stated that the paperwork was getting worse every year. She had to go to work, but wanted to talk some more. She said she goes to a noon AA meeting four blocks from my trailer. She wanted me to meet her there.

I decided to go. The topic that day was on relapse. Three members had relapsed. As they talked about it, I could feel and see the guilt and shame in their faces. When they finished, I spoke the best that I could. I related to them how I went in and out of AA, sober for awhile, then relapsing over and over. The meetings themselves couldn't keep me sober. The meetings were for support. When I realized this, I had to use the 12 step program for recovery. Then I switched stories. I began to talk about my struggle in recovery from my stroke. I had a lot of support; but I knew that I had to do the work, no one could do it for me. In comparison, the struggle with my alcoholism was a piece of cake. In fact, I have been using AA's 12 step program in my stroke recovery. I suggested that they have this group and others as a support system. You have a choice to use it. Get a sponsor to help you with the 12 step program, and let go of all guilt, shame and self pity. These feelings will keep you locked into the path of destruction. After the meeting, a number of members including the three came and wanted to talk some more. This meeting started a series of experiences that put me on the path to help others. The group gave me hope for the future. I continued to go to different meetings, giving and receiving. Something I learned a long time ago is what I get I have to give away, so that I get some more.

The next week, Ginger called to invite me to dinner. Her cousin, Walton and his wife Deborah were there from Washington D.C. I had met them once three years prior at a family party in Fort Myers. I didn't know them very well, but I remember talking with Walton about my profession. I accepted the invitation. It was a wonderful dinner and an enjoyable talk. Then Walton looked into my eyes and confronted me with a question, "What are you going to do with your life?" The question rang loudly in my mind, like a bell that continued ringing. My mouth dropped and I couldn't answer it. He repeated it and added this statement, "After all these years of helping people, now what are you going to do?" Then I uttered these words: I would like to write a book about my experiences with my stroke and recovery in hopes that others would benefit. He basically said that if you can get it together, I will help you get it published.

When I went to bed, my mind was racing, how can I write a book? I couldn't write a book before the stroke. I don't think Walton realized the extent of my brain damage. A part of me was arguing, "You cannot write a book in your condition. Are you crazy?" Deep within me was a spark of energy. Maybe I can, maybe I can get someone to help me. This spark began the emerging of my creative juices.

The next morning, I received a call from another friend whom I hadn't talked to for a year and a half. She had the gift to write. She just called to talk. As we talked, I explained about my idea of writing a book. She seemed excited, then I asked if she would help me. We made a lunch date to discuss how to do the book. The next day I went to meet her. I waited and waited but she didn't show nor bother to call me. I felt disappointed; I didn't even call her to see what happened. I moped around all day, fighting with the part of me who tells me that I can't write a book.

The next day, I decided to run an ad for a ghost writer. I had six responses in the first day. I set up dates to interview each one. I explained my circumstances, followed by the highlights of the story. Each one seemed excited and stated that the book would "fly." Then we had to talk about money, my proposal was to pay them when the book flew. Instead they flew and left me sitting at the table. A few days later a woman responded to the ad. We had lunch, I did my sales pitch, then the money issue, she just smiled. She agreed to help me. Then she took over, the more she talked, I sensed that my book would be hers. She was already changing my experiences. I had fired her before she started.

I decided to let go, maybe I can't write a book. "God's will be done."

The next day I went downtown, wandering aimlessly up and down the streets. I wandered into the "Alley Cat" complex. In the center is a garden, green, colorful, natural and quiet, offering rest to those who lost their way. A place of refuge, prepared by love. As I sat there, I felt a peacefulness in the breeze. As I bathed in the serenity, watching and listening to the songs of the birds, the energy within its very nature seemed to dance, move, create and celebrate. I sat there drinking in the beauty. I noticed a sign at the bottom of a stair case, "Painted Garden." To the left was a painting. I felt the energy emanating from the artist's soul. My interpretation of the painting touched me deeply. It appeared that the artist was in deep conflict within herself.

I sat there for some time, then I decided to leave. As I walked past the stairs, something pulled me back. I went upstairs and I spotted a schedule of art classes, then I walked around the gallery. I met the owner, Kathleen. We talked about the art classes and I found that she was the artist that had created the painting I had admired. I decided to do the classes when I could get some money.

Three days later, I received a call from someone that I had counseled before, asking me if I would work with him again. He had some new problem he was experiencing. I explained my speech problem, but he felt that I could help him. I got off the phone and I called Kathleen. I told her that I wanted to start classes every Tuesday and Wednesday morning. I woke up feeling excited and joyous. I got to the garden early, to feel the serenity. Kathleen had given me a list of supplies to pick up for the classes. I felt like a little boy, sitting there waiting with my paints, brushes, and canvas. Kathleen arrived and told me to look around to find what I wanted to paint. I strolled around the garden. I decided to paint a small part of the garden.

I felt blessed, when I found that I was the only student. I had my easel and canvas in place, brush in hand, ready to begin. I had no clue where to begin. I smiled, she got my message. I knew that I was in the right place. She showed me how to mix the colors, as she finished so was I. My memory deficiencies created a feeling of inadequacy. Again, she was in tune with my energy. We were able to communicate with few words.

Every week I spent four hours in the garden, painting, learning and letting all my limits melt away. It was like a lifting of the barriers of time and space. One morning I brought seven of my completed gourds to the garden. Kathleen put them in her gallery. Now my time was utilized with creating gourds, painting, helping people, biofeedback, yoga, daily reading and Ginger. Even though I still was having problems with my aphasia, eye, and sinuses, when I was in the garden painting, I felt like I had gone to heaven.

The next morning, back in this world, I went to my biofeedback session. I talked with George about my thoughts, which were about balance. This has been my ultimate goal. I have two brains, even though I know that they are connected, why don't I unite them into one power source. My left brain is damaged, which we have stimulated with some success for nine months. I feel that my right brain needs stimulation individually. Then stimulate in the center making oneness.

At this point, I will refer to the Left Brain/Conscious as Jimmy, the male principal and the Right Brain/Unconscious as Muffy, the female principal. We began to experiment with the whole brain and I decided to exercise Muffy more and stimulate her at biofeedback twice a week. My client was doing well in his recovery. A second client made an appointment and an AA member wanted me to help him with the 12 step program. My new life seemed to becoming together.

I had finished my painting, as I sat looking at it, I was feeling excited and elated. I couldn't believe that I painted it. My first painting that I had done a year ago was sitting on the floor. I put my second painting alongside of it. What a difference, from darkness to light. I wanted to show everyone, so I did. I had mixed responses, from "Who cares," "Fantastic," "Wow," "Beautiful," "No comment," and "Who painted it." Immediately, I began another painting. I was spending more time in the garden, just to sit and meditate.

The next morning, I woke up at 4 A.M., feeling peaceful and in a state of balance. I put the coffee on and later I was sitting in bed drinking a cup. I was listening to some relaxing music and my mind seemed very still. I hadn't felt much peace since before my stroke. I had my eyes open, when suddenly, standing at the end of my bed was a hologram. It looked like a scene in *Star Wars*. The image was of a woman that I had met eight years ago. She and I met. Her mother had opened a metaphysical book store called "MoonShadows" in Venice, Florida. I hadn't seen her since the store closed three or four years ago and I couldn't remember her name. She stood there smiling at me. It seemed that I could feel the energy radiating from the hologram. My mind clicked, I remembered that she wanted to write. She had some poetry published a few years ago. Then the hologram vanished. I took a shower and sat there thinking but I couldn't remember where the book store was located in Venice. I knew that her husband owned the building. He had his business in half of it and "MoonShadows" was in the other half. It felt like there was something pushing me. I looked at the clock, a voice in me said that I needed to get there by 11:30 A.M. This was too much.

I went to Venice. I knew the area, so I went up and down the streets. I was feeling discouraged, I still didn't remember her name. I decided to go down one more street and then head back to Sarasota. When I came around the corner, a car pulled into a parking spot across the street. I looked at the driver. There she was. I glanced at my clock, it was exactly 11:30. I rolled my window down, still not remembering her name. My mouth opened, uttering "Cindy!" She looked across the street at me and yelled, "Is that you Jim?"

We went into her office and proceeded to talk. She hadn't heard of my stroke, so I talked about it. She talked about what she had been doing in her life since we had last seen each other. She stated that she had been thinking about me. I hadn't mentioned about my experience with the hologram. She looked at me and stated, "I know why you came here. You want me to help you to write a book." I shared my experiences with the hologram. Cindy wanted to know if I still wanted to write a book about my experiences in the Holotropic Breathwork. I told her that I still wanted to do that book, but this book is about my stroke and recovery. She was finished for the day, so we went to her house to talk about the book.

When we got to the house, I told her about my finances and that I couldn't pay until the book was published. She wasn't concerned about being paid. She stated, "By helping you, maybe I can finish my book that I started two years ago." We decided that if I could tape the story, she could put it together. I felt so excited, I wanted to start now! I went back to Sarasota, I stopped and purchased some blank tapes. My plan was to tape my story over the weekend.

It was Friday, so I thought that I would start it in the evening. I hurried through dinner and showered. I lay on my bed, relaxed myself and began. I turned on the recorder, put the microphone to my mouth. I opened my mouth and became mute. It seemed that my whole story had vanished. It frustrated me, I have a story in my head and I can't express it. Apparently the computer in my head was down. I lay there, listening to my stereo. The music was very relaxing and I fell asleep.

I woke at midnight. I went into the kitchen to get some water. While I was standing there, I focused on my light and sound machine. I went into the living room and browsed through the booklets of programs. I found one that might be appropriate. "YIN-YANG stimulator: 25 minutes, (12–31 HZ). Promotes a link between the Yin (right) and Yang (left) hemispheres of the brain. High Energy." I laid down, put the goggles and earphones on, pushed the button, and proceeded to stimulate my brain.

When finished, I began to tape my story. It seemed to put me into the story because I kept talking, talking and talking to the point that I forgot to turn the tape over. I had over stimulated myself. I listened to the first side of the tape. It was terrible, it sounded like foreign languages. I then went to bed.

On Saturday and Sunday, I taped four tapes. Also, I tried to write, but all I could do was make some short notes and even that took me ten hours. My spelling was out of this world. I listened to the tapes and had to laugh. I couldn't find the words that I wanted to describe how I felt. I hoped that Cindy would be able to use the right words.

Throughout my recovery, I thought that I understood about aphasia. This was the beginning of a long drawn out process of experiences that taught me the true dynamics of aphasia. Speech is a small part of language. Reading and writing are much more difficult. Monday, I went to the garden to paint. I feel so alive when I'm there. I was painting a small statue of a cherub. As I looked at it, I was feeling a sense of being it. I smiled; it appeared as a symbol of little Jimmy. Could my garden, be a symbol of the "GARDEN?" When I finished my class, I drove to Cindy's. I gave her the tapes and notes I made. We talked about the story, she made notes to help her to get into my feelings. She stated that she would do a poem to get herself into the feelings. She suggested that I design the cover. I rushed home, grabbed my paints and began to paint an idea I had in my head. I spent all evening painting. I was proud of my painting. The next day, I drove to Cindy's to show her. She didn't seem excited, so I went back home to rethink my book. I thought and thought and thought until I was going crazy. I decided to let it alone, thinking that it will come by itself in time.

I went to my biofeedback session and told George about writing a book. He just smiled and hooked me up. We stimulated Jimmy first, then Muffy, then united them.

I continued seeing my clients. My yoga classes were helping me on a physical and mental level. My balance was improving, yet many times my balance circuits malfunctioned. Even knowing that I'm fully grounded, my brain sends the message that I'm going to tip over. Consequently a red light will flash, "out of balance, out of balance, tilt, a siren goes off woo, woo, woo." Then my emotional body yells, "We are going to tip over," followed with a feeling of panic. Then many times I grab onto something. It drives me crazy. Rewiring my circuits is a very slow process.

Even though we hadn't begun the book, I was thinking I could have the book finished by Easter of 1995. The days and weeks slipped past. Cindy hadn't written a thing. I was trying to be patient, but after some time, I couldn't help thinking that maybe something is telling me that I have to write the book myself. My heart sunk! I was feeling powerless—How could I write it? I tried to change my thinking, but it seemed like I couldn't. This continued daily.

Cindy finally finished the poem. I thought that it was great, at least we were on our way. My spirits were up. I went to bed excited, joy was racing throughout my body. It took me awhile to get to sleep.

I woke with a start from a dream that had etched in my mind. I sat up in bed to ponder what I had experienced. As I was walking down a dirt road, I came upon a little old woman with a book in her hand. She was dirty and wore rags on her body. It appeared that she had been there for centuries. She had tears running down her cheeks. She asked me if I would buy her book. I took it from her hand to leaf through it, I noticed that the book was perfect. I stated that I never read a perfect book. I asked her why she was crying. She replied "I can't sell it." I said "Why?" She stated "I didn't integrate it."

I didn't know what she meant. Everyday these words kept coming up in my mind. "Integrate it." I knew what the words meant, but not how to apply them.

Cindy had not written a word since she wrote the poem. I talked to her a number of times, asking her how I could help her to help me. She stated that she was busy, but would get on it.

One day I went to the garden, I met a goddess. Many goddesses have come and gone from the "Garden." I knew that some of them dwelled in the spirit world, others dwelled in the concrete world. This was a special goddess; she dwelled in both.

THE GODDESS OF CREATION

I climbed the stairs
to the Painted Garden.
Before me stood a Goddess —
quite gentle in her power.
I greeted her warmly;
She nodded her head in greeting.
I had just emerged from
a long winter of fear.
She reached deep within my soul —
I could feel her vibrations
flowing warmly throughout my body.
Her eyes were tender light
that reflected the colors
of a deep mountain lake.
Her hair reflected a silvery moon
and a golden ray of sunshine.
I dwelled in the mystical light.
Her face was an expression of deepest honor.
I wandered deep within my mind,
struggling to remember.
She brushed my cheek with a gentle kiss __
Her touch was strangely familiar.
I felt that we met many times before —
but I had never seen her until now.
As I was painting —
I could see her, spinning a sense of vitality.

She touched one of the roses —
She seemed to merge with it.
It was beautiful —
Her petals were soft skin.
Her leaves were outstretched arms,
always loving and giving.
Her stem was a source of strength.
A butterfly flitted past —
Butterflies danced around her,
as if she was one of them.
She was the purple mists of evening.
The darkness was
lighted by the shimmery moonlight.
She was delicate, exquisite and rare.
She moved in refined gracefulness.

With her touch, I felt new life
throbbing in my brain and bosom.
I felt new strength, courage, hope and vigor
run through every nerve and fiber in my body.
I was still struggling to remember — .
At last! Ancient memories
began to flood my mind.
She is the Goddess of Creativity.
She is the Goddess of the inner flame.
She is the Womb
of all life and sacred wisdom.
She is the keeper of the fires,
spring, rebirth and inspiration.
Is this but a reflection of myself?
She is warm — she energizes — she creates.
She is ME — I am HER —
She is I — I am She
creating me anew.
We met — we integrated — we are One.
She spoke,
"You may call me when you need me;

I am with you always."

I turned to bid farewell'
The twinkle of her eyes
hung briefly in my inner vision.
All that was left
was her fragrance.

James A. Young
01/01/95

Each time I go back to the "Garden," her fragrance is still there. She was more than a creation of my mind; she exists in my mind. At that moment, I titled the painting that I had just finished; "Eden".

This experience gave me a new strength, courage, vigor, and hope that I hadn't felt before. It helped me to break down the barriers that were preventing me from embarking on a "Mission Impossible."

I had a deep sense that I would have to write my book myself. It scared me, but I was okay with it. I had designed the cover and titled it. Writing the cover story was easy because I could copy words out of my symbol book. Now to find the words and to move them from my brain onto the paper seemed impossible. First, I needed to think about where I should begin. Cindy has the tapes that includes the restaurant, hospital and the first and second weeks at home. Maybe I should start in the third week, just in case she writes the first part.

While I was sitting there trying to write, I became frustrated and stopped. I started to use my left hand, trying to get into a creative mode. After some time, a picture began to emerge. It was an eagle and his mate. He had fallen from the sky hitting the ground. He tried to fly back into the air, and fell into a deep black hole and laid there. I envisioned the words, "Broken Wing." I couldn't spell the words, so I have a small machine called "Language Master LM 4000, a pronouncing dictionary and thesaurus." I tried to write the words on the paper. I couldn't get enough letters into the machine so it couldn't spell the word. It took me twenty minutes to write "Broken Wing."

From this title, and picture I had drawn, emerged a parable. And although it had nothing to do with the book at the time, it turned into the therapeutic emotional catharsis that I needed before I could do the book.

This was the beginning of the "Mission Impossible." To describe my first attempt to write the parable, I invite you to go into my brain, to give you a different viewpoint. You can enter from the back, top of my head, through the soft spot, at which you will meet a guide.

Hi! Please follow me. We will walk forward toward the front. Notice the billions of circuits, connections, antennas, transformers, transmitters, receivers, switches, vast memory banks and highways of wires connected to the central nervous system, in turn, connected to the immune, emotional, and sensory system. I guess the brain is basically a bio-computer, that is a fantastically sensitive instrument with enormous capabilities to reorganize itself and create new pathways.

Notice the past damage, to the left front, that happened thirty five to forty years ago. This damage was caused from extreme alcohol/pot use. Notice that it had been repaired with time, clean air, water, balanced diet and brain exercises.

Look around to the left, notice the new damaged circuits that operate the right leg and arm. Notice the new pathways under construction, causing pain, stiffness, numbness, and clumsiness.

Move a little forward and to the left, you can see the major blast area, knocking out circuits, connections, switches, transmitters, receivers and antennas, damaging others and short circuiting still others. This area has to do with speech and language. Now, look to the big TV monitor, watch Jimmy trying to write this short parable. Notice the time on the clock on his microwave oven, watch the sparks, listen to the hum from his electrical and chemical systems. See and feel the energy produced from his emotional circuits. Some of his systems are not automatic like they used to be. Watch his facial expressions. Look, he's searching for words, listen, Z———, Z———, Z———, he is saying, "Where did all the words go?" The brain is not receiving his question. Look to the right, toward the memory banks, the words are all there, but he has trouble with retrieving them. The communication transmitters, receivers, switches, antennas and memory circuits, received major damage. When he tries to use them, they short circuit. Listen! Look! He got a word, watch his pen move quickly, so he won't lose it. He got it on the paper! Now he is looking at it, Whoa! A sentence came out, he can't write fast enough to get the whole sentence. The end of the sentence vanished. However, he has a number of words, and even though half of them are spelled incorrectly, at least he has a start. Look, watch him use that machine. He can't get enough letters into it to spell the word. Watch his emotions stir! Look at his face! Now he's up pacing. I have to laugh at him, now he's frustrated. He'll be okay, you see, his fires have been lit, and he is no stranger when it comes to frustration. Look at the clock; he's been there for two hours and still hasn't completed a sentence. Now he's looking in the dictionary. He forgets that he can't use the dictionary, his ABC's are all messed up, like a scattered puzzle that had been thrown around the room and pieces are missing. I hope he's never stopped by the police and given the sobriety test where they ask him to recite the alphabet and balance on one leg. They will arrest him on DUI charges.

Oh! I just remembered, I forgot to introduce myself. Hi, I'm Muffy, I am his other half. We have lived together since the beginning of time in this world, so I know him very well.

Now he's back to the desk. Apparently, he gave up trying to use the dictionary. Listen! He's thinking, his inner ears are preventing him to hear some of his thoughts. Sh—"Letly I Ioh haf to rite te stiey ne word at a tom." What he thought was, "Literally, I'll have to write the story, one word at a time." Sh— "It well tic my the rust of my efe." He said, "It will take me the rest of my life to write this book." Now he's crying and sobbing. There is no way that he can write this book without my help. I have connections with spirit. Our relationship has been getting closer and closer, he's been using me a lot. I don't know for certain, but I think it has helped us using the biofeedback equipment. At least, I like it when George wires me up and stimulates me. I'm going to excuse myself, so that I can go down there and help Jimmy.

We continued to write seven days a week, nine hours a day, for two weeks to finish the parable. I was real proud, so I drove to Cindy's to show her. She liked the parable and stated that it could be a child's book. She seemed excited, so she typed it for me. I still hadn't begun the book.

Chapter 16

BROKEN WING

One morning an eagle and his mate were out flying, swooping down looking for something to eat. Suddenly, a shot rang out, echoing throughout the mountains. The eagle fell to the ground. Dazed and in shock, he laid there in disbelief. He tried to get up to fly back into the air, but his right wing was broken and shattered. His mate flew down to help him, but she was powerless to do anything to help him. As she watched him lie on the ground, she could only cry. She knew that she had to get back into the air for her own safety. She watched helplessly, knowing all she could do was try to protect him, the best way she could. They both knew that he was prey on the ground. His wing lay lifeless, he became afraid and anxious, because he couldn't fly. He tried to get back up in the air, but it was no use. His mate came down many times to protect and feed him. She wanted to stay with him, but she knew she could not, for she needed to get back to the nest.

It was a very long and lonely night. He longed to be able to fly once again with his mate. He could not feel his right wing, and blamed it on the cold night air. Alone and feeling abandoned, he didn't know if he would ever fly again. His mind wandered as he thought back to how in one moment he went from a powerful, free, courageous, spirited eagle, to a powerless, fearful, and trapped eagle. Feeling threatened about his survival, he struggled over and over to fly, but it was dark and he felt tired. He decided to rest and try again tomorrow.

In the morning, a Shaman of great knowledge appeared before the eagle. He told the eagle he could fix only the broken part of the wing. The eagle would have to fix the shattered part of the wing himself. He was the only one that could heal that part of himself. The Shaman called him "Broken Wing," and gave him an herbal potion to drink when he felt strong enough. The Shaman picked Broken Wing up and laid him in the weeds to heal. He explained that Broken Wing would be safer in the weeds because no one would see him there. Broken

Wing struggled everyday, trying to get back into the air. Everyday his mate came to watch over him and protect him through his struggle. She came even though it meant risking her own safety. They both knew how vulnerable Broken Wing was on the ground. When a predator would come close, his mate would distract them and fight to protect him. Days, weeks, and months passed as Broken Wing began to heal. He still could not fly. Every time he tried, his right wing would give him much pain. He had also damaged his eyes in the fall. He was also feeling very unbalanced, so sometimes when he stood he would tip right over. He remembered the Shaman's message, and in time he got stronger and was able to defend himself. Now his mate would not have to risk her life by coming to the ground. Struggling everyday to get back in the air left Broken Wing exhausted.

Months passed, then Broken Wing took sick. His mate came to care for him, but there was not much she could do. Broken Wing just lay there very still. He could not eat and was getting weaker. He feared he would never fly again. So one night when his mate was not near, he got up. He was very unstable and passed out. Just as a predator was about to kill him, his mate swooped down and saved him. As time passed, Broken Wing slowly got better. Again he tried to fly. This time he made it off the ground, only to fall into a black hole. His mate could see him, but was unable to reach him. Broken Wing was stuck in that hole for weeks. He tried many times to get out, but couldn't. He was trapped. As his mate circled in the air watching him, she could see him struggling, but could not help him. This left her feeling sad and frightened. She began to fly higher and higher, so she didn't have to watch him struggle. Broken Wing felt frightened and anxious as he watched his mate disappear in the sky. He mustered all of his inner strength and was able to free himself from the black hole where he had been trapped. As time passed, he was forced to learn to take care of himself on the ground. His mate had to continue with her own survival. She had flown so high, Broken Wing could not see her anymore. He was sad because he could not fly with her. He missed her immensely, and it hurt him to see her go. He remembered all the times they flew together, exploring the world. One of his young ones came down to the ground, she helped him build a nest there, so he would be safe.

One day his mate appeared, she had returned to see the nest that he and the young one had built. Her eyes were sad. She told Broken Wing that she was about to fly off to another part of the world. Once again he was hurt, because he could not fly with her. He continued his healing, and was beginning to feel more integrated and balanced. At last Broken Wing took flight.

Some say that you can hear in the wind, "I can fly . . . I can fly."

Others say that Broken Wing is half eagle, half man. The eagle flies at night, the man is on the ground today!

Chapter 17

THE ACUPUNCTURE AND HERB DOCTORS

   Meanwhile back in the "Garden," I had completed my painting. My pride welled up inside me so I had to run around and show my painting to everyone. One morning when I was at the "Garden," Kathleen mentioned that her husband, Andy, had just finished school in acupuncture. I thought that maybe he could help me with my sinuses and the muscles around my right eye. I made an appointment and met Andy. I felt totally comfortable with him and sensed a spiritual connection. Even though he was newly licensed as an acupunturist, I felt a level of instant trust that I cannot explain. My intuition was strong that I was in the proper place and time, as if I were being touched by a very dear and loving old friend of 100 years acquaintance. I didn't understand totally the dynamics of how acupuncture worked, but I knew the method was holistic, based on the idea that no single part can be understood except in its relation to the whole. The theory is based on two polar complements, Yin/Yang, (Male/Female). They are convenient labels used to describe how things function in relation to each other and to the universe. Also, they represent a way of thinking. This system of thought considers each as parts of a whole. The principle is to transform them into each other. When the two principles are out of balance symptoms will appear.

   The theory is that working with points on the surface of the body and using needles to stimulate the energy, will in turn affect what goes on inside of the body. Accoding to the book *The Web That Has No Weaver*, the points are on what they call meridians. "Meridians are the channels or pathways that carry Qi and blood through the body. They are not blood vessels, rather, they comprise an invisible network that links together all the fundamental substances and organs." "Qi is the energy associated with movement (any movement)."

   I told Andy about my stroke. He could see that I had trouble with my speech, but I told him what I wanted fixed, my immune system, sinuses and the muscles around my right eye.

He examined me by way of feeling my pulse and looking at my tongue. He stated that I was having a problem with my liver and my wind. I couldn't understand about wind, other than as the outer wind, that affects me and makes me agitated. I understood about the liver. I was aware that at birth I was jaundiced and that they thought I was going to die. Then I thought about all the alcohol that I drank. That sure didn't help my liver. Andy stated that maybe the liver started the process of having my stroke. He couldn't be certain if it had.

I laid on my right side and he put needles in the area of my head where I received the brain damage. Then he put needles around my sinuses and around the muscle of my eye. He also put needles in the area of my liver and around other areas. I had a small problem with the needles. It didn't hurt, but my eye seemed super-sensitive and when he put the needles around it, I became very agitated. After a while, I became comfortable. I laid there listening to peaceful music and went to sleep.

When I was finished, Andy recommended that I take herbs as part of the treatment. I called the herbalist, Patrick White and I was able to see him that day. I told him about my stroke, but I didn't tell him that I had seen Andy. He examined me by way of feeling my pulse and looking at my tongue. He also told me the same thing. That I had a problem with my liver and my wind. He stated that the liver problems could have caused my stroke.

He uses natural herbs, so I watched him bag up all of the different herbs, a handful of this, a handful of that. It appeared as if he had raked his lawn, dirt, bark, sticks, weeds, flowers and grass. He put the cooking directions on the bag. I envisioned myself cooking a witches brew, outside on an open fire, in a black kettle, with a black hat and cape. I chuckled to myself.

I had scheduled two acupuncture treatments twice a week. Unbelievably, Andy refused any payment except for the needles, about $5.00 a session. I drank herbs, twice a day, seven days a week. After a while, I was noticing that the treatments were helping. I was able to get off the Afrin. My eye improved considerably, so I continued receiving treatments.

It was the first of June 1994, two years since the stroke. I came to realize that I had to write the book myself. I called Cindy and went to Venice to get my tapes. I felt disappointed and angered because I couldn't seem to find someone to help me. I thought, "God! Haven't I had enough? Give me a break." I continued to think about it, then realized that maybe there is a reason for this and it will show itself later.

I decided that I was going to stop painting and creating gourds for awhile. I wanted to continue with the Biofeedback and acupuncture on Tuesdays and Thursdays, so I scheduled them back to back. I scheduled my clients on those days so not to lose much time. I knew that it was going to be a big job for me to write a book.

Chapter 18

THE WRITER

All my experiences, sensations and impressions were so vividly etched on my mind that I couldn't possibly forget them. There was nothing wrong with my mind. The pictures were clear and colorful, strong and powerful. Remembering each occurrence was akin to many human experiences that are never forgotten: the sound of a barking dog; the image of a rainbow; the smell of wood burning. But how could I possibly write about it? How could I convey the emotion and anguish?

How should I do it? Before my stroke, I could type eighty words a minute. At that time it was automatic, my thoughts would go down my arms and into my hands, hitting the keys. Now typing was no longer an automatic process. The interrelation of my arms, hands, and the typewriter keys no longer existed. The memory loss of the letters on the keys, plus the lack of proper brain signals to strike the correct keys made it impossible to type. I decided to use a pencil with an eraser.

I listened to the first tape. I tried to write what I had said, but I had tremendous difficulties putting the words on paper. To describe how it works, the brain controls all of the complex events required to speak, write and understand language. We don't think about it, because it's automatic. We just write or speak, but when your brain is damaged it is not an automatic process.

Step 1.   We have to think about what we want to communicate.
Step 2.   We have to put the thoughts into words.
Step 3.   We have to keep the words in our head until it is spoken or written.
Step 4.   The message goes down the arm and out of my pencil onto the paper.

At times, step 1 gets lost or my inner ear cannot hear the thoughts.

Consequently it stops the process, then I have to start over to find the thought. Sometimes I cannot find it. Sometimes I can get step 1 and go into step 2 and actually get some of the words, only to lose them; then I have to start over. Sometimes I can get through steps 1-2-3, but the message won't go down my arm and out my pencil onto the paper, then I have to start over. Sometimes I can go through steps 1-2-3-4, and the message goes onto the paper backwards, or the spelling is so bad I can't read it. Sometimes the message gets on the paper perfectly, but when I read it back, it doesn't seem to be right, so I change it.

I committed myself to write everyday, no matter how I felt, until the book was completed. I had no idea how to convey my story, I thought that I would just write what I had experienced. I hoped, trusted, and had faith in Spirit to guide me through the process.

I had no conscious idea of what I was doing. I remembered what I had learned about how sounds affect the energies in the brain and body. I decided to see if sound would help me to write. I filled my CD player with classical music, the uplifting type, Mozart, Bach, Chopin, Beethoven, and one CD with Chakra music. I put my earphones on, as I was sitting there listening and breathing, it seemed to pull my inner energies together. It seemed like there was a silent pulse of rhythm within.

I started to write, literally, one—word—at—a—time. I was able to get myself back in time and feel as if I was there, re-experiencing the events. Words would come up and I would try to field them, like a baseball center fielder. Some words I would miss, others I would drop, but at times, I was catching a few. I put the words on the paper. I circled each one, then I would associate other words and connect them, until I could construct a phrase, then sentences. It was like a 10,000 piece puzzle, connecting each piece together to get the total picture. I found it frustrating and interesting at the same time.

At times, Muffy would create humor out of the frustration. Other times she would laugh and be silly. In turn we escaped the barriers of time and space. When we were tired, we slept, only to return with a new found energy. This went on twenty-four hours a day, seven days a week for the whole month of June.

I continued to write daily, and I began to notice that my writing was starting to improve. One night I went to bed early because I was tired, but I woke up having a tremendous anxiety attack. I wasn't aware of having a dream, it seemed to just happen. There was no rational reason for it. It was at 1:00 A.M., Sunday, I flew out of bed, pacing back and forth in the trailer. I tried breathing. I tried lying down. That was worse, so I paced and paced trying to breathe it away. In time it had lessened a little, but I couldn't lay down. It felt like I was spinning around and around. On two occasions, I was going to wake my neighbor, but I didn't. It seemed like I couldn't get it under control. Because I couldn't, my mind seemed to race and race out of control. I waited until it was 7:00 A.M., then I went to my neighbor's trailer.

I talked and talked releasing some of my pent up energy, until it seemed to lighten me up. I was worried about my blood pressure so at 9:00 A.M., my neighbor drove me to WalMart to use the blood pressure machine. It was excellent, 130/80. That made me feel better, so we went home and I went to bed.

I got through the episode and was feeling good. A week passed. One morning at 2:00 A.M., someone was knocking on my door. I opened the door. My neighbor, the woman who had the stroke, was standing there in shock. She came in and stood there in a trance. I knew something happened, so I asked what it was. She kept looking at me, then she tried to speak, but because of her stroke, it was very difficult for her. From what I could understand, her husband died. Apparently she had just come from the hospital. She began to cry, chills ran up and down my body. He was fifty-six years old and I had talked with him a couple of days ago. He sounded and looked good at that time. There she was, trying to deal with her stroke, now this. I comforted her and listened to her express her feelings the best she could. After awhile, she went home.

A few days later, I came down with the flu. Oh! No! My mind went right back to the time in my early recovery, it scared me to death. I called to cancel my appointment with Andy. He stated that he would come over and give me treatments and special herbs to help me get through my sickness. Laurie came and helped every day. Ginger brought healing chicken soup. I really felt grateful for those three, all I could do was lie there in bed, hurting. When I get down, whether I am sick or just tired, my speech and language skills regress. I believe that the love from Andy, Laurie, and Ginger, plus the treatments, herbs and soup, got me through my sickness in a week.

I recovered and felt good. My speech and language skills came back where they were before and I continued to write. After some time, I noticed that I was in total frustration. I struggled, working all day with no productivity. Then I realized that I wasn't using my music or Muffy. When I did, it made a difference.

My life had become a world of isolation, with the center being writing, with a sprinkle of biofeedback and acupuncture. In a sense, it was a positive thing, but on the other side, I needed to have some outer stimulation to get a balance. I had quit yoga, but now I decided to go back.

Chapter 19

THE BRIDGE

On October 30, 1994, I had a vivid dream, the kind that I have that gets etched in fine detail in my mind, and that I can't forget.

It started in my hometown. I was standing on the corner when a beautiful blond female drove up in a Volkswagon Beatle and rolled down the window. She smiled, showing her beautiful white teeth that sparkled in the sun. She asked me if I wanted to go with her on an adventure. Of course I couldn't refuse, so I jumped in and as she drove down the road, I asked her where we were going. She replied, "I don't know, but it will be an exiting experience. She drove to the next town and parked in a no parking spot and asked me to keep the engine going so she wouldn't get a ticket. Then she went into a department store. After some time, a cop came by and warned me to get the car out of there, so I drove around for some time, waiting, which seemed forever. Finally, I spotted her and drove around the block. She had a hundred people with her. I stated that there isn't enough room for everyone, she smiled at me and told them to get in anyway. They all got in, I cracked up with laughter. She jumped in next to me and I continued to drive.

We drove out of town on a new eight lane highway. Down the highway we came to an intersection, with numerous roads branching in all different directions. I stopped and asked which road. The blond stated, "straight ahead," so I continued to drive. As we got out into the country, the road turned into a paved two lane road. The country was beautiful with lush green grasses and beautiful colored wild flowers and stands of trees. The road was a hilly, winding, curvy road that meandered into the distance.

We came around a curve and there was a huge gorgeous home nestled into the hill. Some of the people wanted to stop, so I went up the driveway. Half of them got out and stated that they wanted to stay there, because they were afraid of where the road would lead them.

So we went back to the road and continued our journey. Down the road the same thing happened, half of the remaining people got out and stated that they were afraid. So we went back to the road and continued on our way. Again it happened, everyone got out including the blond, I stopped her and asked: "Why? You wanted me to go with you on this adventure. Get back in the car." She wasn't smiling anymore and she looked frightened. I stated that I came this far, so I have to go on to find out where this road leads to.

I drove out of the driveway and onto the road. I looked back, she was standing there waving, with tears dripping down her cheeks; I felt sad because I didn't get to know her. I headed down the road feeling all alone. I kept driving and driving thinking about when I was going to get there. Then I climbed a steep hill and as I went around a curve, I looked into the distance—there it was. It was a majestic bridge that went into the clouds; it had a deck as wide as a fifty lane highway. It appeared that it was under construction, there were hundreds of roads that came into it. I drove down the hill to see where it led. When I got there, there were some barriers in the way and a stop sign, that said "Under Construction." I crashed the barriers and drove along the side of the bridge, going up and down the piles and mounds of dirt, crossing huge ruts. I climbed until my vehicle stopped. I was so excited I got out of my vehicle, picked it up and put it underneath my arm, continued to climb the side of the deck still hanging onto my vehicle. I couldn't believe the size of the deck as I climbed onto it. I walked to the edge into the clouds, I have had some highs in my life, but this was the highest I have ever experienced. I walked still hanging onto my vehicle. I looked down to see a huge river meandering through the forest. A huge eagle was flying in front of me looking down at the river. I looked down to see what he was looking at. I saw hundreds of salmon struggling to get up the stream. Along the edge and out around the landscape were huge lights. It looked completed, except for the landscaping. Huge power equipment vehicles were working. I wanted to jump the gap. I could see the grandeur on the other side, but I had feelings of fear in my stomach, so I got into my vehicle and drove off the deck and went back to the hill to view it some more. I camped there on the hill, waiting patiently. As I was sitting viewing the stars, the "Voice" said "DO NOTHING"—I woke up still hearing the words "DO NOTHING."

That morning, I went to my Bio-feedback session having an anxiety attack on the way, thinking that I would not get there. George wired me up and I was still hearing the words, "DO NOTHING," so I did nothing. I didn't even look at the screen, but I could hear the feedback ringing in my ears consistently. When I was finished, George looked at the graph, it was excellent. He stated, "What did you do? Whatever it was, keep doing it." I smiled at him and stated, "I DID NOTHING." He looked at me and smiled as if I was joking. I had not told him of my dream and decided to keep it a secret for awhile to see if something else would come up for me. I went back home and started researching some of the symbols that were in my dream in one of my favorite books, *A Dictionary of Symbols* by J. C. Cirlot.

Using this book, I was able to interpret my dream. In the dream, I left home (my birth Home) with a partner, and one hundred individuals. When we got to the intersection we had to make a choice. My partner made the choice and everyone agreed to go straight ahead. I view the road, as the "Road of human life."

When we found the first Home, some decided to stop there, because it was a comfortable Home and they didn't want to take a risk of finding another. When we found the second and third Home, the remainder decided to stop there. I decided to go all the way.

All the roads coming into the bridge were symbolic of "All roads lead to God." The barriers on the Bridge were barriers that I had built to stop myself from finding God.

The Bridge symbolizes the union of heaven and earth or link between what can be perceived and what is beyond perception or transition from one state to another.

The River corresponds to the creative power, both of nature and of time.

The Eagle symbolizes the spirit or the struggle between the spiritual and celestial principle and the lower world. The eagle plays the role of a messenger from heaven and is regarded as the most apt expression of divine majesty.

The Fish is a psychic being and the symbol of the fish represents the life-force surging up. For instance, salmon are born in the mountains and take a journey from the mountains to the sea and then try to find their way back to their home; against all odds, struggling against the current, and leaping waterfalls, they find their home and create new life. As soon as salmon spawn, they die. The eagles and bears feast on the dead salmon and the salmon gives life-force to them.

The Lights are traditionally equated with the spirit. Light is also the creative force. Psychologically speaking, to become illuminated is to become aware of a source of light and in consequence of spiritual strength.

The Trees, with their roots underground and their branches rising to the sky, symbolize an upward trend.

The Volkswagon was my body. It seemed to me, the dream was a preview of where I was heading and to erase any fear that I had.

I continued writing. My neighbor was having trouble dealing with her grief, so I suggested that she write her feelings on paper. She stated in her jumbled up speech that she couldn't write. I smiled and stated that I can't either. A few days passed and she came over with a few pages of writing. She gave them to me expecting me to read them. I gave them back to her and stated that I can't read, so I want you to read it to me. She began to do the best she could; as she read out loud, her emotions moved out of her body, and she cried and sobbed. When she was finished, she looked brighter. She thanked me and went home. She stayed away for a couple of weeks. One day, she came over to show me two poems that she wrote. She read them to me, they were excellent. She continued writing poems and kept a journal, and she joined the "Naked Poetry Society" where they read their poems, naked. (Joke). Through the months that followed, I noticed that it was helping her with her recovery.

This Thanksgiving, I felt in touch with the true meaning of the word. I got up at 5 A.M. As I was sitting at my desk, playing with words, I had no idea that I was creating a poem. As I was putting the words on paper, they seemed to flow together. When I finished I had a beautiful Spiritual poem.

At 10 A.M., I went with Ginger and her son Phillip, and his wife, Susan, to Fort Myers for Thanksgiving dinner. The whole family gathered on the farm. The weather was ideal, so we ate outside beneath the old oak trees. To me it looked like the first Thanksgiving with the Pilgrims and Indians gathered together.

I was grateful for being alive. I had gratitude because my speech, writing, and language skills improved. I could walk, run, and dance. My anxiety problem was improved. I created a home out of nothing for myself. My creative self had been emerging outward to this world. My physical balance had improved and I was feeling a closeness with Ginger. Ginger and I stayed with her mother. Phillip and Susan stayed with Ginger's brother, Rick. I like staying at her mother's because I get up early and watch the sunrise come across the river, greeting the new day. As the darkness merges into the light, everything comes alive.

Throughout December, I had several anxiety attacks while I was sleeping. I knew they were coming out of my subconscious, but I didn't know what they were connected to. The only thing I could do was to trust and have faith in spirit to show me.

Some friends of Ginger's and mine wanted us to go with them on a Christmas cruise to Mexico for five days. I was broke, so I couldn't go. Ginger decided to go with them, so just before Christmas, Ginger and I went to Fort Myers for an early Christmas dinner and gift exchange. To watch the kids, made my day. Rick's little son, Ricky, who resembled me as a young child, had designed, drawn and colored a Christmas card in art class. He won first place in the contest throughout the school. Rick had it printed so they could send it out for Christmas. He was so proud and I could see his little eyes were sparkling and his little soul was emanating out into the room. This year's Christmas sure beat last Christmas. Maybe my life is finally turning around.

New Years Eve, we had a few of our friends over for a New Years Eve party and dinner. It was a wonderful and enjoyable party. I was so grateful, especially when I thought about last year's holidays. Also I hadn't had an anxiety attack for a week and a half.

The next morning, we got up to a beautiful day, had breakfast, and went for a walk. It was one of those days that you totally appreciate, peace, joy and happiness. Around two, I had decided to go home to write, I kissed Ginger and Lucy good-bye and went to write. I wrote all the rest of the day.

Around seven in the evening, Ginger called; when I heard her voice, I felt a deep feeling of love towards her. What a day and I was feeling so good. We talked for awhile, then it happened. She stated that she called to tell me that she wanted to be honest with me. She had a new boyfriend. I knew it before this time, but I thought that it would go away. She said that he was coming to stay with her for three weeks. BAM—I went into shock, followed with feelings of fear; then I went into pain, then into anger, then back to fear, followed with severe pain in my heart. This all took place in a minute. I went from heaven to hell. I stated, "Don't ever call or come over, like you did a year ago, I am very angry and underneath it is a lot of pain, because for a year I have been receiving double messages." I hung up and it felt like she stabbed me with a long blunt knife that went into the center of my heart and out of my back. I grasped my last breath, staggering toward my bed to die with my boots on. As I lay there, still with no struggle, I died.

I got up the next morning and began to write, I never thought about her again. I just wrote and had anxiety attacks.

Chapter 20

REBIRTH

Throughout the process of writing, I relived, felt and integrated my experiences into my psyche. I had become more and more aware of the whole. However, a big piece of the whole was missing. I had a major block in my emotional and psychological bodies.

I noticed it sometime ago, my anxiety attacks were different, they happened in my sleep. I would wake-up in them, usually in early morning. There was no rational reason for them. They had begun to increase in terms of time and severity. It came to a head in mid-January. I talked to numerous people, but I still couldn't figure it out.

One day I was seriously thinking about getting some Xanax. My life seemed pretty good except for the anxiety attacks. I was beginning to think that I would have this problem the rest of my life. I called a friend and told him of my dilemma. He stated that, "You have gone this long without using drugs, something will come to you." He also stated that he remembered me telling my clients, over and over, when they were in a crisis and feeling overwhelmed that "God won't give you more than you can handle." Now I had to eat my words.

I started to have flashbacks of a new born infant; my physical body would tremble, shake and twitch. This happened on three separate days. The third day it happened, I was lying in bed and I realized that I was re-experiencing my original birth. At this point, I need to explain about how I know about my birth. I will share my first experience with rebirth. About seven years ago, I started to do what is called Holotropic Breathworks, the Greek words *holos*, meaning "whole" and *tepein* meaning "moving toward." It is a very powerful, safe, tool to use to get into altered states of consciousness. It was founded by Stanislow Grof, M.D, Ph.D. I won't describe how to do it, because you shouldn't do it without an experienced person with you. In the back of the book, I will give you the addresses to get information.

I went to workshops at least once, sometimes twice a month for a year, then sporadically for four years. This tool has helped me to become more and more aware of myself in relationship to the whole. At times I was able to experience beyond the brain, into a higher mind, where everything that I, as soul ever experienced.

Holotropic Breathworks is done in a group. The first thing you do is pick a partner, called a "sitter." The sitter acts as a caretaker and provides human contact. The breather lies down on a mat. The idea is not to go into it with an agenda, but to let go and let spirit choose the experience. If the breather gets into an altered state and into the experience, then usually another part of himself called the "observer self" comes and observes. It is there so that the breather can see what's happening and at the same time he is actually back in time where the event was taking place. In this case, I was actually being the baby.

I had no trouble letting go and after awhile I started to feel a lot of anxiety in my present body. Then I was the fetus. My mother was in labor and she was about to propel me out of the womb. Instead of struggling like normal babies to get out of the womb, I resisted. It looked like I had both feet braced so I couldn't be birthed. Then my mother pushed out. I came out so fast, I felt like I was a bullet.

In the experience, I heard myself say "I'm not ready;" but I was moving so fast my umbilical cord ripped causing severe pain in my adult body. At that time I envisioned that the doctor grabbed it and pulled it out by the roots. (Note, after the experience my adult body hurt for over a week). There I was lying on a cold steel table, my little body looked about nine inches tall, and I was totally yellow and in total shock. I didn't cry, it was like my emotional body had shut down. I started to feel cold and then it felt like I was freezing to death, but no one was helping me. In the experience, my adult body passed out; as the baby, I woke up in an incubator.

I couldn't believe what I had experienced at this Breathworks. So the next day I called my father and asked him what details he remembered from my birth. He told me I was a six month baby, totally yellow and that I was so little I could fit into his palm of his hand. The doctor had told him that I would surely die. This was the first time that I had heard this about my birth.

I have only been admitted into a hospital twice in this lifetime. The first was my birth, the second was my stroke. Apparently my stroke triggered old memories from my birth. I believe now, that I was having my stroke on the way to the restaurant. When we passed the hospital going to the restaurant, the strange feelings I had and the knot in my stomach were memories from my birth. The tremendous anxiety that I was having at dinner was from both, my birth and the stroke. When I went into the hospital, my anxiety decreased because I went into shock, and when I felt like no one was doing anything to help me, that was coming from the memories of my birth. When I was feeling like I was freezing and when I was sensing that the hospital and doctors were going to kill me, and when I wanted to run, that was memories of my birth. When I had to go back to the hospital to get my records and when I went to visit Jose, my anxiety attacks were from my birth. When Ginger told me about what the psychic told her, when I was in Perry, the anxiety attacks were from my birth.

All the experiences when I had trouble breathing were from my birth, coupled with my three near-drownings I had when I was a small child. I was reliving the suffocation experienced at birth. In a sense, I had five serious brushes with death, creating issues of survival and impermanence.

On the behavioral level my life has been that of survival rather than living. I had a stormy sense of impermanence, wandering around the country seeking and searching for my Home.

The vision of my ego encased in a suit of armor was his fear of death; as he sensed the impending threat to his dissolution from his position of power, he fired the first shot that started my inner civil war.

The tremendous resistance that I experienced through my recovery was both from the brain damage and from my birth. Resistance/surrender is the process of letting go. My ego, through the biochemistry of fear, was battling for his life. For two and a half years, my ego raged on slowly losing his power.

After this revisit of my birth, I went back through my entire life and wrote a searching and fearless personal inventory, especially the experiences I had while doing Holotropic Breathing. I could see the complete whole. At this time, I choose not to share it because it is another book in itself.

As I continued to write this book, I sensed the completion was coming closer. I hadn't talked to Ginger for the month of January and I hadn't thought about her. On February 2, 1995, at four P.M., I was driving to the grocery store, all of a sudden, a surge of energy rushed into my head, Ginger was standing there in my inner vision, it was like something turned on my inner TV—the screen was very clear and in color. The date and time were displayed in the upper right side of the screen, I don't know why.

I felt a deep feeling of emptiness move through my body as tears ran down my cheeks. I parked in the parking lot at the store and sat there to compose myself. My inner TV was still playing, so I turned it off, as I was walking towards the store, a part of me turned it back on. I turned it off again; again it was turned back on. This conflict continued throughout my shopping and on the drive home. When I arrived home, I sat there crying tears of emptiness and tears of love, not feelings of sexuality but a deeper inner spiritual love. I didn't like the empty feelings, but I sure liked the spiritual connection.

I turned on my outer TV in the hopes that I could drown out this image and feelings. To feel the strong spiritual connection was beautiful, but the emotional and mental connection was hell. She was my best friend, lover and everything that I had seen as a special relationship. I knew that I had to let go of her on the physical, emotional, and mental level and to transmute the feelings. But I didn't know how.

I had dinner and went to bed to watch outer TV. After awhile, I was tired and found myself nodding off to sleep. It was only nine P.M., but I turned off the TV and laid down to sleep. In five minutes, my inner TV was playing loudly, I tried everything to turn it off. This went on until ten and finally I went to sleep.

I awoke at one A.M. feeling an inner coldness. It seemed like I was freezing inside. My body was shaking and trembling outwardly. I got up and put my heater on, and then I went back to sleep.

When I awoke, I had a cup of coffee and sat in bed pondering my experience with the cold After relaxing for awhile and listening to some music, my mind took off and took me back to revisit my birth for the third time. Visions were presented to me, like movie clips. The themes were about abandonment and the pain and anxiety of separation.

To feel abandonment is to feel deserted by God or to lose sight of the light. My birth and my life were filled with separation and abandonment. My perception at birth was that God, mother, father, and the doctor abandoned me leaving me enraged at life and this world. Later the movie continued to show numerous close relationships that I had in my life. Every relationship ended in abandonment. As I looked at them, I could see that the special relationship isn't outside of myself, but the special relationship is within the union of God, Ego/Spirit and Muffy/Jimmy, flowing in harmony. I felt that I got in touch with the true meaning of the words, "Marriage Made In Heaven." Another positive note is that the inner Love relationship won't abandon me.

After this experience, I felt drained, so I went back to sleep. I began to dream a dream that was so real, it was spooky. The cast was me, Ginger, three males I knew and one male I didn't know and a male I hadn't met, but who I knew because of his accent. The dream gave me some answers to questions that were bothering me for some time. (Note, at this time, I choose not to share this dream in detail.) I can say this, Ginger and I have a lot of ancient history, in turn I have a strong spiritual connection with her. I don't have to be with her on a physical level. These experiences seemed to lift my anxiety.

I continued writing and could see the end was near. Going into April, I had to declare bankruptcy. It seemed as if I finally let go of all of my attachments that I had in the physical emotional and mental bodies. What I had experienced throughout the process was a form of purification. My bridge has finally been completed that leads to union in myself. I see spirit as the bridge. My special relationship is born within me.

In the "Garden," Man/Woman, originally had the same power. The union of feminine and masculine energies within is the basis of all creation. Female intuition/Male strong action equals creativity. The female aspect, is the intuitive self and is the deepest and wisest part of me. Maybe some of you have heard of the saying, "Behind every Great Man, there is a Great Woman." Reconnecting with the inner feminine power, enhances and strengthens my masculine qualities.

I now believe that if it wasn't for Muffy, I couldn't have written this book, when you have left brain damage and aphasia, it is impossible to write a book.

Creativity is synonymous with Spirit. Creation is synonymous with communication. Wholeness is synonymous with reconciliation of opposites. "When I cannot communicate with my inner man or woman, I can't communicate with the physical men and women with which I must interact." The circle of creation has no end. It's starting and it's ending are the same. In itself it holds the universe of all creation, without beginning and without an end.

My completion hinged on the decision to listen to the "VOICE."

THE VOICE

An ancient memory haunts me ——
I don't recognize —— THE VOICE ——.
THE VOICE reminds me ——
This world is not your home!
As if there were — a place
That calls me to return.
I'm in exile here — and feel, alien.

A persistent feeling — causing me
To walk the world,
In an endless search.

I seek in the darkness,
THE VOICE whispers,
Of my home.

"Where is my HOME?"
I whisper back.

In that instant, —
THE VOICE, ——
Takes me HOME in perfect stillness —
My HOME is silent and in peace,
Beyond all words, and untouched
By fear and doubt ——.

James A. Young 01/07/95

I believe that the world of bodies (Ego) is the lowest world of all creation and that there isn't a hell or death. Death is an illusion. Death is Ego's Fear. Most people are programmed to fear God. The word Death scares everyone. Now I believe that the word Death means freedom, leaving, a passage, a surrendering into LIFE. The word Death is a very positive thing. Joy and freedom arises from the knowledge that death is an illusion.

The idea that loss is possible is insane; I can't lose anything, because I never had it to lose.

The world of bodies trying to merge with each other keeps the illusion of separation alive.

The world of bodies is backwards and upside down and is the opposite of Heaven.

Ego/Body are the same, my Ego separated my Soul from its real form and subjected it to the cycles of births and rebirths.

My Ego had put his claws into my mind and heart, and Ego had entangled my Soul in passions, anger, fear, greed, attachments, lust, and vanity. I wrote a short poem titled Edging God Out.

Edging God Out

My body draws a circle
Infinitely small around a
small segment of Heaven.

Splintered from the Whole
proclaiming, that within it,
Is my Kingdom.

Within this Kingdom,
My EGO rules cruelly,
Edging God Out.

Like a tiny ripple on

The ocean surface,

On a tiny sunbeam, to the Sun,

Each tiny fragment,
Seems to be self-contained,
Needing the whole to give it meaning.

Alone and frightened—
Holding me apart from the universe.

Let go of my body,
With its tiny senses—
So that I can see the
Grandeur that surrounds Me. ——

James A. Young
11/25/94

I am not an Ego, I am not my body, I am my Soul. The very fact that I can do what I have done, and bring any order into chaos, shows me that I am not an Ego, and that more than an Ego must be in me. For the Ego is chaos, and if it were all of me, no order at all would be possible. I have POWER to choose—I have POWER to learn—I have POWER to change viewpoints—I have POWER mightier than EGO. The POWER of His Will.

I embraced His gift of death in order that I could live.

Chapter 21

SPIRIT IS THE ANSWER TO SEPARATION

When my ancient journey began, the end was certain. Doubt and despair only came to go, and went to come again. I didn't know that my path was circular, so I walked and walked, round and around, going UP to the mountain tops, DOWN to the valleys of shadows, DOWN into the swamps. I finally noticed that I kept seeing familiar landmarks wherever I went, then I realized, I never actually left HOME—The JOKE was on me, as GOD laughed, "Oh! Oh! Oh!—My SON, my SON you journeyed hard and courageously. Heaven is not a place, nor a condition. It is merely an awareness of perfect ONENESS and the knowledge that there is nothing else, nothing OUTSIDE of this ONENESS." One healing brightness, a pure and Holy PEACE, envelopes me and holds me safe in pure lovingness in the MIND of GOD.

Now I know, that I do not walk alone, for GOD is here, NOW, he has always been with me. I didn't listen to the VOICE, I allowed, believed and listened to KING EGO. I thought that I had LOST my way, but what I found was the meaning of LIFE. The stillness and the peace of NOW enfold me in perfect gentleness—Everything is gone—except the Truth:

> Spirit, being a creation
> Of the ONE creator.
> Spirit, is the answer
> To separation.
> Spirit brings King EGO to GOD.
> Spirit abides in MIND.
> Spirit will prevail
> This is MY TRUTH. I don't know what your TRUTH is.
> Only you do.
> I can't give it to you. You are RESPONSIBLE

My rebirth will last forever, I go out and meet my newborn world. I arise OUT OF THE ASHES. I go in FAITH, knowing that God guides me and all I have to do is NOTHING. I celebrate my salvation on this Easter morning, April 16, 1995.

I have reached the END—or is it the Beginning?

Chapter 22

TRAGEDY or BLESSING?

Where there had seemed to be no Life, no possibility of development and no power, a new and powerful Life emerged, out of the ashes.

As I sifted through the ashes, it became clear to me what this was all about.

I believe that my Spirit taught me through comparisons and used opposites to point the way to my truth; it had to do this because opposites gave me an awareness of the only power I had left: The Power of choice. It's ironic, or is it? Spirit teaching me in this way, this was the way I taught my clients. The first thing I would do was discuss the dynamics of choice. From their responses, I could get a picture to see where to begin. Most had no idea that they even had choices. When they grasped the dynamics of choice then they got better, because they took responsibility for themselves.

Spirit gave me struggle, sorrow, pain, grief, depression, anxiety, despair and persistence. They were devices to force me to respond to the law of change. In the second day in the hospital, I chose the quest for wholeness and I turned my will and life over to God. So actually, I asked for this not knowing what it was going to involve. Because I didn't know, it put me into a position to exercise my faith and trust in Spirit. I was hoping that I would get a big miracle, but instead I experienced numerous smaller miracles.

Once I chose, I had a "burning desire" to get better and a "willingness to go to any length to get it." I had a positive attitude, somehow I was able to hang on to it throughout the process. I believe, now, that it was directed from Spirit and supported with a cast of many. Many extras were used, and were placed along my path without their knowledge and directed on cue to cross my path and to give me the pieces that I needed to get me better.

The second step required action; struggle is action. Birth or Rebirth involves struggle to have Life. I have gained from my struggles. First of all, I gained an awareness that I was able to reach into my Soul and found powers available for my use. Powers I never knew I possessed. Without persistence, I never would have discovered them. If you ever noticed, the tallest and strongest tree stands alone. The reason that it's tall and strong is because it is in constant struggle with the wind and elements.

Persistence seemed to arouse my enthusiasm and inspired my imagination. Without struggle, the fulfillment of my "Mission Impossible" wouldn't have happened. Neither would I have been able to learn that what seemed impossible, by taking action proved to be possible. Writing this book gave me a therapy beyond my imagination. It moved me to discover even more about myself; it also helped improve my speech and language skills, my communication and opened new mediums to express myself. Struggle produced the birth of still another medium: poetry. I had heard that poetry is the language of the gods. It is like music, melody and rhythm. I believe that this is true; poetic form can be seen in history, Lincoln's Gettysburg speech, The Declaration of Independence, The Lord's prayer, and Sermon on the Mount.

On Thanksgiving day this year, 1994, I wrote my first piece of poetry. In my experience, when I write a poem it seems to release a flood of energy within me; I realize that this is spiritual energy. It seems to enable me to overcome fatigue and adversity. Writing poetry gives me orgasmic experiences; sometimes it is better then sex.

Now, I believe, that expression is a need similar to water and food. To be able to express myself positively in many mediums helps open and keep open my spiritual channel. When I block my emotional and mental energy, the flow of energy has to go somewhere. So it will manifest in many ways. Some of it is manifested in sickness, anger, depression and behavior. To be able to express myself in many mediums helps my energy to flow smoothly.

The emotion of sorrow is a true humbling experience; without it, I wouldn't have recognized Spirit. It broke down the barriers that I had set up or permitted others to establish in my mind. They stood between my physical body and my spiritual potential. When I broke down these barriers, I felt a freedom that I never had known.

Sorrow can be a curse or a blessing. It's the negative side of a human emotion and can become self-pity. I discovered many years ago that self-pity is one of the most destructive feelings I have. It drains my positive energy. At times in the early part of recovery, I was feeling that my sorrows were greater than I could bear. Each day when I awoke, I had a choice, so I would relax and pray to God to get me through this day so I wouldn't get into self-pity. At times, I would stray into it, but I was able to get back out of it.

Sickness and suffering, is it a misfortune or a blessing? Is it stumbling blocks or is it stepping stones? It all depends on one's perception or view. Its always your choice. I was able to perceive it as a blessing, so I took advantage of the situation. I didn't like some of the choices, but I had a deep sense that God had to be there with me each step of the way, because the amount of distress that I was creating in myself would have blown me apart.

Pain put me in a position to practice letting go and turning it over to Spirit. Because I didn't like the pain, I had to choose to let it go. I rediscovered how I create everything that I experience in life, no one does it to me. I am responsible to deal with anything that I experience. For example, I didn't want to let go of Ginger; consequently, I was creating all of my pain, myself—she didn't create it for me.

In April, a friend I hadn't seen for a couple of years stopped over to the trailer. She noticed the name "New Moon" embedded in the front of the trailer. She asked if I had known the meaning. I honestly didn't know. She stated, "New Moon represents the release of inhibitors. The New Moon favors releasing and flushing away these critical inhibitors that block us from manifesting our good. All old patterns of being and anything that does not serve us should be released at the New Moon." Ironically I had been releasing my old patterns as I struggled to make the trailer my home. The depression that I created was the beginning of the process of giving up or losing of the old self and was an integral part of the process of my mental and spiritual growth. Actually it was a normal and basically healthy phenomenon. I chose not to use drugs to stop the process, consequently I had a beautiful experience of letting go and was able to see the shadow side of God.

Fear, poverty, sorrow, pain, misery, over anxiety, worry, anger, frustration, unpleasant circumstances can be transmuted into inspirational forces of good benefit.

The major lessons I was given are about creativity, death/life, letting go, patience, judging others, and love; consequently because of these lessons, I discovered and rediscovered other pieces of knowledge.

On the physical level, my right side is still numb, but it doesn't hurt and it's not tight anymore. My eyes are okay and they don't give me any trouble. My sinuses are okay and my immune system seems to be working normally. I haven't had any sickness and I don't have allergies anymore. My balance has been restored and I haven't had to grab onto anything.

My brain is still in the process of creating new pathways. It has created a lot of new paths thus far. I guess at this level, where the energy is heavy, it takes time. I don't know if I can explain what numerous people have asked me, how can you write a book and still have aphasia?

My aphasia is still a daily problem. From what other stroke survivors, who have ten to thirty years of recovery, tell me, it will cause me trouble maybe for the rest of my life.

My speech and writing abilities have improved a lot because of what I have done. My speech goes up and down. I can talk to you at times and you won't know that I have a problem. If we sit here for fifteen minutes and talk, it's like my batteries seem to run down. It depends on what I am doing or how I am feeling. Fatigue, stress, the feeling that the world is going too fast, and even when I'm calm and relaxed, my electrical system just doesn't work at times.

I repeat sentences as if I hadn't said them. When I write a note, I mess up the spelling. For example, Bonnie called and gave me a number. I wrote Bobbie instead of Bonnie and the number was incorrect. Two pages ago I wanted the word slurring of speech, I wrote sluffing of speech. Sometimes I can't listen, process, and write all at the same time. I can only pronounce a few technical terms or foreign names and my spoken vocabulary is minimal. When I write, I can take time to find the words; even if I have to, as I did, reread the pages a hundred times. When I speak, however, I can't take that much time. Aphasia is now just a part of my life and me. I guess for some you can't explain; not unless they could switch brains for a day. A friend in the stroke club told me that every Saturday she goes to the bar and drinks cokes and talks to drunks. They understand the speech. I can believe this, because that's what it's like. In fact, many people with strokes have been misdiagnosed at the emergency rooms and have been told that they are just drunk.

My emotional body seems clean. I haven't had any anxiety attacks, pain, grief, depression, or sorrow. What I have been experiencing is an inner happiness and joy that doesn't depend on outer stimulation. When I do go out, it goes with me and I have peace and serenity. I feel like a child at times and have the childlike spontaneity. I love it. With the old farts, it's a problem; so I guess I'll have to hang around with the young people.

I have no resentments or regrets; I see that my stroke was a blessing. I'm still me. I still enjoy life and I love everyone. I never had seen Ash Wednesday, Palm Sunday, and Easter like I see it now. Out of my ashes, I celebrate Palm Sunday and celebrate my victory and acceptance of my truth. I am happily in the celebration of LIFE. Easter is a sign of peace. I gave Ginger and me a gift of lilies to celebrate a time of joy.

The weekend of Easter, I started to exercise my typing skills. I found that I still have trouble reading the directions and understanding them.

It took me a day to get the screen up on the word processor so that I could begin typing. When I began typing, my right arm, hand, and fingers gave me trouble. After awhile, my fingers began to stiffen up and my arm and hand would move to the right and my fingers would be on the wrong letters.

The next day, I was able to type a long poem for Ginger that I had written a week prior.

Then it took me forever to figure out what keys to push to make it print. My neighbor came over and helped me and it got done.

I decided to continue exercising my typing skills, so I put this on my recovery program.

The Friday of Easter, I had been invited to speak at an open AA meeting. The other speaker was a colleague of mine who had worked with me at "Genesis Center" in Doctors Hospital here in Sarasota. I hadn't seen him in two years.

I was the first speaker. And although I felt nervous at first speaking to approximately 100–150 people, when I stood up in front of the microphone, it went away. I said, "I am Jim and I am an alcoholic," and they yelled "Hi Jim!," then I was able to stand there and to talk with few problems for twenty-five minutes. I felt like I was connected with every person in that room.

We in AA do not judge each other and it felt so wonderful to be accepted as I am. For the last three years, I've never had so many people judge me because of my speech in all my life. Because of it, I will never judge my brothers and sisters for the rest of my life. An old Indian said:

DO NOT JUDGE AND
CRITICIZE YOUR FELLOW
MAN, UNTIL YOU
HAVE WALKED IN
HIS MOCCASINS FOR A MILE.

Also, my gourds have been selling at the "Painted Garden."

My journey followed a route which is the inverse of that path which I took when I entered into it on October 4, 1937. My path took me to my creation. I found the secret of my truth, so I wrote the following poem.

TRUTH

The Truth is hidden,
Deep within, under a
Heavy cloud of Fear, that
Manifests in many forms.
The cloud is dense
and obscuring
Reach in, beyond the
Dark and heavy cloud.
Go through it, to
THE LIGHT
My strength is not my own
That gives me power.
God is my source

James A. Young
4/6/95

AFTERWORD

We have been taught that by exercising regularly, eating a balanced diet, staying away from alcohol, drugs, and cigarettes we will live longer.

I believe this, but most people don't think about their brains. You can have a gorgeous body that is healthy, but when you ignore exercising the brain, you will lose it, then you can sit around with your beautiful body in a stupor.

I believe that the brain is like a muscle like any other muscle. It needs exercising. Researchers, Scientists are beginning to understand that the brain has a remarkable capacity to change and grow. Recent research suggests that stimulating the brain with mental exercises may cause brain cells, called neurons, to branch wildly, causing millions of additional connections, or synapses between brain cells.

We have two brains. Exercise both.

* * *

All of life should be a learning experience in order to have a healthy brain. It has to be challenged, if challenged it will build brain circuitry. Brain exercising can be a fun thing.

Using math problems, drawing, writing, reading aloud, practice meditation, and focusing attention on an object. You should check out the book *Brain Power* by Vernon H. Mark, M.D. FAC.S. with Jeffrey P. Mark, M.SC.

Do puzzles, crosswords and or a jigsaw puzzle. Musical instruments, dance, the Arts can be a powerful vehicle through which to challenge the brain, stir creativity, instill discipline and build self-esteem.

At this time, I need to state that research demonstrates that there is a connection with the brain and immune system. The brain and immune system communicate with each other. Brain damage interrupts communication with the immune system, and also there is a bond between the immune and the nervous system that seem to be even more intimate. They also found that the left brain has the more direct influence on the immune system.

I see Thomas A. Edison as a man who used both of his brains. He basically hypnotized himself to enter into his subconscious and beyond, and found his secrets. I quote Mr. Edison, "The only reason we need the body is to carry the brain around. The brain is dominant." "If we did all the things we are capable of, we would literally astound ourselves." He had ten thousand failures, or you might see it as successes, before he found the secret of the light bulb.

I found in my total experiences in the last twenty-five years and its support with research, that beyond the brain exists, quite apart from the structure of the brain, a mind with an enormous capacity. This mind is a powerful entity; it never loses its creative force, it never sleeps, it creates at every instant. There are no idle thoughts, all things produce form at some level. This mind is naturally abstract. God communicates with his creation, this communication is perfectly abstract since its quality is universal in application.

The human body, is a part of the mind that had split and become concrete. Ego depends on the concrete.

INFORMATION AND SOURCES

INFORMATION AND ADDRESSES OF HOLOTROPIC BREATHWORK
ALCHEMICAL HYPNOTHERAPY AND BIOFEEDBACK RESEARCH

Grof Transpersonal Training: To learn more about Holotropic Breathwork or about how to become a certified practitioner, contact:
Grof Transpersonal Training
20 Sunnyside Ave., Ste A-314;
Mill Valley, CA 94941
or call (415) 383-8779

Jacquelyn Small
Eupsychian Press
950 Roadrunner Road
Austin, Texas 78746

Alchemical Hypnotherapy Institute
2310 Warwick Dr.
Santa Rosa, CA 95405

Biofeedback Research Paper
George Rozelle, Ph.D.
2477 Stickney Point Road
Sarasota, Florida 34231

SOURCES:

A Dictionary of Symbols
Second Edition by
J.E. Cirlot & Jack Sage
Routledge & Kegan Ltd, London 1962
published by philosophical Library, Inc.
200 West 57th Street, New York, NY 10019

Alcoholics Anonymous
Third Edition, Twenty-fifth printing 1986
Copyright 1939, 1955, 1976 by
Alcoholics Anonymous World Services, Inc.
Box 459, Grand Central Station
New York, NY 10163

Reverend Alex Orbito
Psychic Surgeon
Manila Phillipines

The Web That Has No Weaver: Understanding Chinese Medicine
Ted J. Kaptchuk O.M.D.

Super Memory: The Revolution
Sheila Ostrander and Schroeder

Memories, Dreams, Reflections
Random House 1973

Brain Power
Venon Mark and Jeffrey Paul Mark
Houghton Mifflin Co.
2 Park St.
Boston Mass.

Strokes: What familiesShould Know
Bruce B. Grynbaum
Ballantine Book Division of Random House Inc.
New York

In the Shadow of the Shaman
Amber Wolfe
Slewellyn Publications
St. Paul, Minn. 55164

Transpersonal Psychotherapy
Edited By Seymour Boorstein, M.D.
Science & Behavior Books Inc.
701 Welch Road
Palo, CA 94306

Jung's Quest for Wholeness
Curtis D. Smith
Published by State University of New York Press
Albany, NY

The Way of the Shaman
Michael Harner
A Guide to power and healing

Science of Breath: A Practical Guide
Swami Rama
Rudolph Ballentine, M.D.
Alan Hymes, M.D.

The Art of Breathing and Centering
Gay and Kathlyn Hendricks
The Hendricks Institute
P.O. Box 994
Colorado Springs, CO 80901

A Course in Miracles

Published by the Foundation for Inner Peace
P.O. Box 1104
Glen Ellen, CA 95442

Hands of Light: A Guide to Healing Through the Human Energy Field
By: Barbara Ann Brennan

ABOUT THE AUTHOR

He was born in Chippewa Falls, Wisconsin, on October 4, 1937. He was raised there until the age of seventeen, then he joined the U.S. Navy. After his discharge, he went back to Chippewa Falls and worked there until age forty-two. He then obtained employment in Kalispell, Montana and stayed there three years. Then he obtained employment in Sarasota, Florida, where he still resides.

All his life, he had a burning desire to answer this question, "What is life?" This world for him, seemed backwards and upside down. He had a deep sense that this world wasn't his home. What he was taught contradicted the behavior of his teachers. They talked about love, but the behavior was hate. In his hunger for the truth, he took the path of shaman.

In his quest, he was introduced to the spirits, (Alcohol) at a young age. The spirits lifted him to a new height and he felt that he had found the answer, he could do almost anything—as long as he was drinking. When the alcohol turned on him, he quit drinking. This was when he realized that he needed more knowledge. In 1972, he began to work with alcoholics and drug dependents and he became a pioneer in the recovery field and a new paradigm thinker and teacher. He felt that this was his calling.

In his thirst for knowledge, he returned to the Catholic Church, looking for answers. Not finding the answers he was looking for, he moved from church to church, religion to religion, picking up knowledge as he went.

He found in nature, part of the answer. He always felt very comfortable and secure there, as if this was his home. Throughout his quest, it seemed that nature pulled him back from time to time to get renewal. As he continued his quest, he studied the writings of Carl Jung, Edgar Cayce, Abraham Maslow, Alfred Adler, William Glasser M.D. and Carl Rogers. He practiced Reality, Gestalt, and Transpersonal therapy and he is an alchemical hypnotherapist.

On his journey, he found Eckankar, the ancient science of Soul travel, he was able to relate well with the writings of the founder Paul

Twitchell. He explored the churches of Metaphysics and The Science of Mind.

From there he began to study the Eastern and Western mysticism. He tried to study Quantum physics, but it is still a mystery to him. However, it changed his perception by looking at the human body as nothing more than pure moving energy with different vibrations. He also studied the Chakra energy system and practiced manipulating the energy with breath and sound.

He has a spirit of adventure like "Indiana Jones" and a willingness to risk using new techniques and modes to explore the inner mind. He gets his aspirations from great men in history that went beyond the brain, such as Thomas Edison and Bill W.

Twenty five years ago, he began his career in the helping profession; even then, he believed in wholeness. He worked in hospital based programs and found a conflict of beliefs. Way back, they came up with the disease concept, so most programs were called the medical models. He became a maverick and took his beliefs underground and operated there.

About four and a half years ago, he took a position at Anabasis Inc., a private treatment center for Chemical Dependence.

He took the position because the staff had the same beliefs that he had. The owner, Peg Buzzelli was also a maverick in her own right. They were experiencing the same conflict with the medical model. So he felt that at least he wasn't all alone and he could then come up out of the underground.

The staff met once a week and complained about the increasing paper work and how much time they were spending fighting with insurance companies. There was a decision to write a new paradigm, the old, had to die. It took about a year to write the new paradigm and was finished in June 1992.

His future looked rosy, his life was on track, he had a wonderful active relationship, an active social calendar, a private counseling business that was becoming prosperous and he was in good health.

FROM THE AUTHOR! BOOK COVER STORY

The book cover was a birth in itself. One day while I was trying to design it, I closed my eyes; I was concentrating on creating an image on the screen of my mind. My mind was a blank. I sat there in silence. Then I realized, I was using my left brain. If I need a design, then I needed to access my creative self, which resides in my right brain and expresses herself through my left hand. I put my pen in my left hand, and began to scribble. After some time, I opened my eyes. It appeared to be a kindergarten art class picture, full of scribbling. I threw it in the corner of my living room in disgust.

For about two weeks, I struggled with the design, without success. One day, I was looking up the meaning of a word in my symbols dictionary, I opened the book and saw a symbol that looked familiar. I focused my attention on the kindergarten art work, that I had tossed in the corner. There it was.

The symbol is called a Mandorla, an almond shaped figure formed by two intersecting circles. The Mandorla symbolizes the intersection of the two spheres of Heaven and Earth. The two circles have come to be regarded as the left, Matter (Ego) and the right, (spirit), life/death, powerless/power, and conscious/unconscious. These words and concepts are attempts to express an experience or knowledge of the union, bringing together or being brought together into an integrated whole. The flame in the center symbolizes transcendental upon the environment.

The blue at the bottom of the flame represents water. The Chinese consider that life comes from water. Water is the beginning and the end of all things on earth. Alchemists gave the name of "water" to quicksilver, in its first stage of transmutation and by analogy, also to the "fluid body" of man. This fluid body is integrated by modern psychology as a symbol of the unconscious that is of the non-formal dynamic, motivating, the female side of the personality. By analogy, water stands as a mediator between life and death, with a two-way positive and negative flow of creation and destruction.

The fire in the Egyptian Hieroglyphics is an expression of spiritual energy. The alchemists' and heraclitean notion of fire was the agent of transmutation, since all things derive from and return to fire. Fire, just like water, is a symbol of transformation and regeneration. There is a Hindu image representing the joining of opposites (analogous to the marriage of fire and water, by the interlocking of man and woman.)

Ashes are considered capable of stimulating growth of the cornfields and well-being of man and animals.

The back of the cover is the first attempt of designing it. Actually, I painted the end of the book first. It has been standing in my living room throughout the writing of this book. As I was writing the end, I realized, It is the end.

It represents the center of my being. My ego had been defeated in my inner civil war and my self (spirit) takes its rightful place as the center of my psyche, thus, the self is resurrected.

In the center is creation, on my human dimension, the egg and the sperm unite, emanating the colors of the chakras system in the body. Also in the center and beyond is the "Garden" where pre-separation took place.